Women's Wellness
Navigating Your Health Journey

Kevin D. Harper

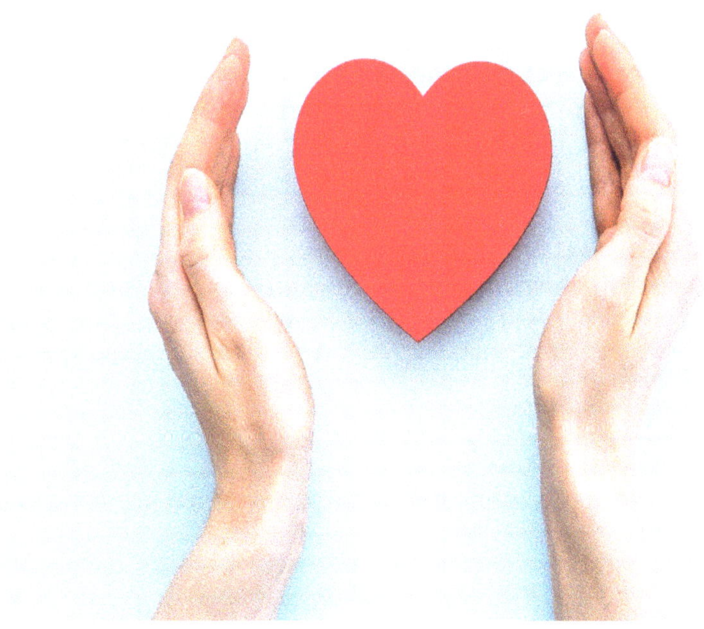

Copyright © by Kevin D. Harper

Introduction

Welcome to Women's Wellness: Navigating Your Health Journey. This book empowers women with the tools, knowledge, and confidence to take charge of their health and well-being. Every woman deserves to live her healthiest life, and understanding your unique wellness needs is the first step toward achieving that goal. Whether you're navigating physical health, mental well-being, or emotional balance, this guide will provide essential insights and practical advice for women of all ages and backgrounds.

Women's Wellness is about more than just trends in a world filled with conflicting information and quick-fix solutions. It's about building a sustainable, holistic approach to well-being rooted in research, self-care, and personal empowerment.

What You'll Discover Inside:

- **Comprehensive Health Insights**: Learn about key health issues that women face, including hormonal balance, reproductive health, and preventative care.

- **Mind-Body Connection**: Learn how mental health, emotional well-being, and physical fitness are interconnected and how to nurture each aspect for a balanced life.

- **Practical Wellness Strategies**: Discover actionable tips on nutrition, exercise, stress management, and self-care practices that fit your lifestyle.

- **Empowerment and Self-Care**: Learn how to prioritize your needs and create a wellness plan that aligns with your goals and values.

Why This Book Is for You:

- **If you want to understand your body better**, explore how different life stages impact women's health and how you can support your body's changing needs.

- **If you want to improve your mental well-being**, discover practical strategies for managing stress, anxiety, and emotional health.

- **If you're ready to take control of your health journey**, empower yourself with knowledge, guidance, and the confidence to make informed decisions about your well-being.

Women's Wellness isn't just a guide; it's an invitation to transform your life by taking small, sustainable steps toward lasting health and happiness. Let's embark on this wellness journey together.

Are you ready to navigate your health journey with confidence? Let's get started!

Table of Contents

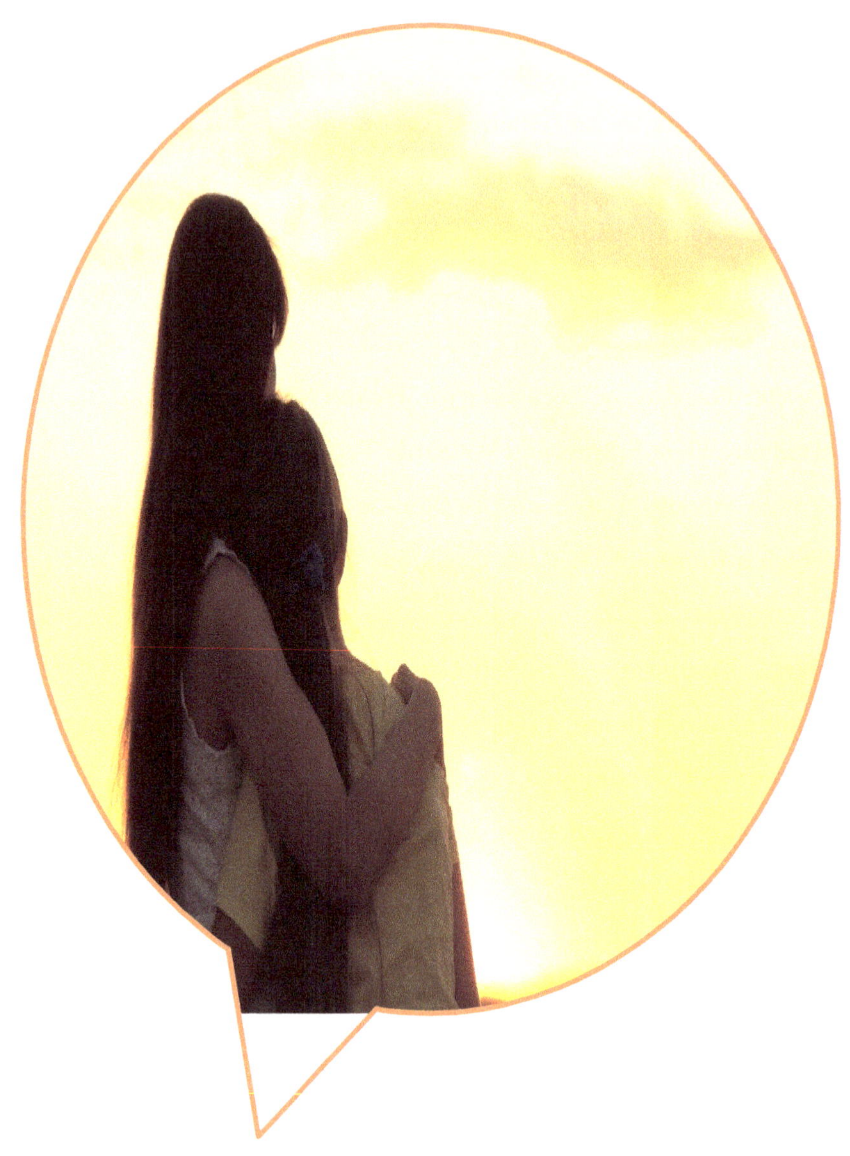

Women's health is a vast and dynamic field of study that focuses on understanding the unique medical, physiological, psychological, and social aspects of women's lives. The health challenges women face are varied and often intertwined with their biological differences, life stages, and social roles. As women tend to live longer than men, their health needs change over time, and they must navigate specific health issues that require attention to both prevention and treatment. A clear understanding of women's health is crucial not only for practitioners in the medical field but also for society as a whole, ensuring that women receive adequate and informed care.

1.1 Overview of Women's Health and its Unique Aspects

1.1.1 Biological and Physiological Factors

Women's health is influenced by biological and physiological factors that make their health needs unique. From puberty to menopause and beyond, women undergo a series of natural processes that impact their health. For example:

- **Hormonal Changes:** Women's hormone fluctuations significantly impact women's health, especially during puberty, menstruation, pregnancy, and menopause. Estrogen, progesterone, and other hormones influence both reproductive health and bones, cardiovascular systems, and mental health.

- **Reproductive System:** Women have specific reproductive health concerns, including menstrual health, pregnancy, childbirth, and menopause. Issues such as polycystic ovary syndrome (PCOS), fibroids, endometriosis, and fertility problems are common in women and require targeted medical attention.

- **Immune System Differences:** Women generally have stronger immune responses than men, but they also face a higher risk for autoimmune diseases like lupus and multiple sclerosis, which may require unique treatment strategies.

1.1.2 Life Stages and Their Health Implications

Women's health can be divided into various life stages, each presenting specific health challenges. These stages include:

- **Adolescence (Puberty):** During puberty, girls experience rapid physical and hormonal changes, which can result in challenges such as menstrual irregularities, acne, and body image issues. These factors can affect their mental health and overall well-being.

- **Reproductive Years:** During this stage, women may face challenges such as contraception choices, pregnancy complications, and menstrual disorders. Gynecological issues like ovarian cysts, fibroids, and cervical cancer are concerns that become more prevalent during this time.

- **Pregnancy and Childbirth:** Pregnancy represents a unique aspect of women's health, with risks ranging from gestational diabetes to preeclampsia and complications during labor. Understanding maternal health and ensuring the mother and baby's safety is crucial.
- **Menopause and Post menopause:** As women age, they experience menopause, the cessation of menstruation, which comes with its own set of health issues. Menopause is often accompanied by symptoms such as hot flashes, mood swings, and osteoporosis. Postmenopausal women are at a higher risk for cardiovascular diseases, bone fractures, and certain cancers.

1.2 Importance of a Holistic Approach to Health

A holistic approach to health means recognizing that health is not just the absence of disease but a person's overall physical, mental, and emotional well-being. For women, a holistic approach considers all aspects of their health and recognizes the interconnections between their physical, emotional, and social environments.

1.2.1 Physical Health

While women's physical health is essential, it is closely tied to their mental and emotional states. Chronic stress can result in physical ailments like high blood pressure, while poor nutrition or lack of exercise can exacerbate mental health conditions. A holistic view ensures that these dimensions are considered together.

1.2.2 Mental and Emotional Health

Women's mental health is just as important as their physical health. Studies show that women are more likely to experience mental health conditions such as anxiety, depression, and eating disorders than men. These mental health issues often correlate with hormonal fluctuations, social pressures, and life stresses unique to women. A holistic approach ensures that mental health is not overlooked, especially during key life transitions like pregnancy, postpartum, and menopause.

1.2.3 Social and Cultural Influences

Social and cultural factors also influence women's health. These can include family and community roles, economic status, access to healthcare, and exposure to violence or discrimination. In many societies, women face barriers to accessing healthcare due to financial constraints, gender-based discrimination, and cultural expectations. A holistic approach to women's health considers these socio-cultural determinants, ensuring that healthcare delivery is sensitive to the unique challenges women face.

1.2.4 Preventative Healthcare and Lifestyle

A holistic approach also emphasizes the importance of preventative healthcare, including maintaining a healthy lifestyle, eating a balanced diet, exercising, and managing stress. Preventative care for women includes regular screenings, vaccinations, and counseling on topics like sexual health, mental well-being, and managing chronic conditions like diabetes or hypertension. By focusing on prevention, many diseases and conditions can be managed more effectively before they become serious health threats.

1.3 Common Health Issues Faced by Women

Women face a broad range of health challenges that are either exclusive to them or more common among them than men. These conditions are often rooted in biological differences, but they may also be exacerbated by societal factors such as access to healthcare, mental health stigma, and work-life balance.

1.3.1 Reproductive Health Issues

Women's reproductive health is an area that encompasses a wide array of conditions and concerns. Some of the most common reproductive health issues include:

- **Menstrual Disorders:** Problems like heavy periods (menorrhagia), painful periods (dysmenorrhea), and irregular cycles are standard among women of reproductive age. Conditions like endometriosis and PCOS can also cause menstrual irregularities.
- **Infertility:** Infertility is defined as the inability to conceive after one year of regular, unprotected intercourse. Both men and women contribute to infertility, but women's issues like blocked fallopian tubes, hormonal imbalances, or ovulation disorders are common causes.
- **Pregnancy Complications:** Pregnancy can present numerous health challenges, including gestational diabetes, preeclampsia (high blood pressure), and high-risk pregnancies requiring specialized care.
- **Cervical and Ovarian Cancer:** Cervical and ovarian cancers are among the leading causes of cancer-related deaths in women. However, they are often preventable with early detection through regular screenings such as Pap smears and HPV vaccines.

1.3.2 Cardiovascular Health

Heart disease is the leading cause of death for women worldwide. Despite this, heart disease is often under-recognized in women. Women tend to have different symptoms of heart attacks than men, making diagnosis more difficult. Moreover, hormonal changes during menopause can increase a woman's risk of cardiovascular problems. Some risk factors for heart disease include high cholesterol, high blood pressure, obesity, and smoking.

1.3.3 Osteoporosis

Osteoporosis, a condition that weakens bones, is more common in women than in men, especially after menopause. Estrogen plays a crucial role in maintaining bone density, so the drop in estrogen levels during menopause significantly increases the risk of fractures. Women with osteoporosis often experience breaks or fractures, even from minor falls.

1.3.4 Mental Health Issues

As mentioned earlier, women are more likely than men to suffer from mental health issues such as depression, anxiety, and eating disorders. Societal pressures, hormonal fluctuations, and experiences like childbirth and menopause can all contribute to mental health conditions. Additionally, women are more likely to suffer from conditions like post-traumatic stress disorder (PTSD), often linked to experiences of violence, abuse, or societal trauma.

1.3.5 Autoimmune Diseases

Autoimmune diseases like rheumatoid arthritis, lupus, and multiple sclerosis disproportionately affect women. The immune system mistakenly attacks healthy cells, leading to inflammation and tissue damage. The cause of these diseases is not fully understood, but hormonal, genetic, and environmental factors play a role in their onset.

1.3.6 Sexually Transmitted Infections (STIs)

Women are more susceptible to certain sexually transmitted infections, including chlamydia, gonorrhea, and human papillomavirus (HPV). Regular screenings, safe sexual practices, and vaccinations like the HPV vaccine can help reduce the risks associated with STIs.

1.3.7 Menopause and Perimenopause

Menopause marks the end of a woman's menstrual cycles and fertility. It typically occurs around 50 but can happen earlier or later. Symptoms include hot flashes, night sweats, mood changes, and changes in sexual health. Osteoporosis and heart disease risks increase after menopause, making healthcare monitoring crucial during this period.

1.3.8 Urinary Tract Health

Due to the shorter length of the urethra, women are more prone to urinary tract infections (UTIs), which can be recurrent and cause significant discomfort. Urinary incontinence is also a concern in older women, and it may be related to childbirth, aging, or pelvic floor disorders.

Conclusion

Understanding women's health is essential for improving care and outcomes for women at every stage of life. By recognizing the unique aspects of women's biology, taking a holistic approach to health, and addressing common health issues such as reproductive health, mental health, and chronic diseases, healthcare providers can better support women in achieving optimal health. Women's health is not a singular issue but a complex interplay of biological, emotional, and social factors that require nuanced, thoughtful care.

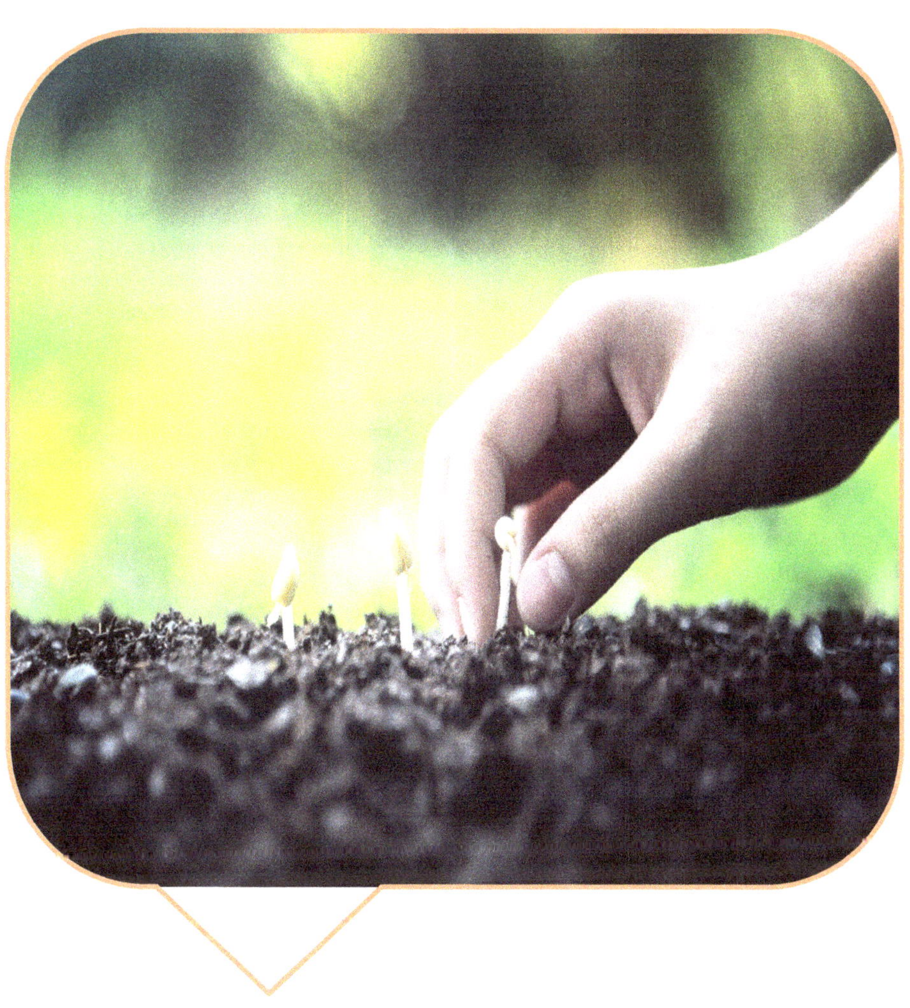

Introduction:

A woman's life is characterized by developmental stages with distinct physiological, emotional, and health-related transitions. These stages include adolescence, the reproductive years, menopause, and the postmenopausal phase. Understanding each stage's changes and health considerations is crucial for maintaining overall well-being. This chapter will explore these life stages in detail, providing a comprehensive view of how a woman's body and mind evolve and what healthcare considerations are paramount at each stage.

1. **Overview of Different Life Stages**

A woman's life can broadly be divided into four main stages: adolescence, the reproductive years, menopause, and beyond. Each stage is associated with unique physical, hormonal, and psychological changes that influence a woman's health, lifestyle, and overall well-being.

Adolescence (Ages 12-18)

Adolescence marks the transition from childhood to adulthood. This stage is often defined by rapid physical growth, sexual maturation, and emotional development. Puberty, typically occurring between 8 and 13, develops the reproductive system. Key milestones include the onset of menstruation (menarche), breast development, and the growth of pubic and underarm hair.

- **Physical Changes:** In addition to sexual maturity, adolescence is marked by the development of secondary sexual characteristics, including increased body fat, widening of the hips, and changes in skin texture. Growth spurts are common, with many girls reaching their adult height by the end of this phase.

- **Psychological and Emotional Development:** This stage is also characterized by the search for identity, emotional volatility, and the development of social relationships. Peer influence becomes prominent, and there is a growing desire for independence from parents.

Reproductive Years (Ages 18-45)

The reproductive years are marked by the peak of fertility, typically from late adolescence to the mid-30s. This stage is associated with regular menstruation, the ability to conceive, and various physical and emotional changes related to childbearing.

- **Fertility and Menstrual Cycles:** During this stage, a woman experiences regular menstrual cycles, typically lasting 28 days, with hormonal fluctuations governing the cycle. Ovulation occurs around the middle of each cycle, which is key for conception. Regular periods and reproductive health are central concerns during this stage.

- **Pregnancy and Childbirth:** For many women, pregnancy is a significant part of their reproductive years. This stage involves a profound set of physical and emotional changes as the body prepares for and supports the development of a fetus. Hormonal changes support fetal growth, increase blood volume, and modify the cardiovascular and respiratory systems to accommodate the pregnancy.

- **Postpartum Period:** After childbirth, a woman's body undergoes recovery and adjustment, both physically and hormonally. Postpartum depression can also affect emotional well-being during this time.
- **Contraception and Family Planning:** Women in this stage often engage in family planning, managing contraception, and making reproductive decisions.

Menopause (Ages 45-55)

Menopause marks the end of a woman's reproductive years and is characterized by the cessation of menstruation. It typically occurs between the ages of 45 and 55 and signals a major hormonal shift, particularly the decline of estrogen and progesterone levels.

- **Perimenopause:** This stage typically begins several years before menopause and is characterized by irregular menstrual cycles, hot flashes, sleep disturbances, and mood swings. Women may experience fluctuating levels of estrogen and progesterone, which can lead to irregular periods and other symptoms such as vaginal dryness and reduced libido.
- **Physical Symptoms:** The decrease in estrogen levels during menopause can have profound effects on the body. Hot flashes, night sweats, weight gain, changes in skin elasticity, and thinning hair are common. Osteoporosis and heart disease risks increase as estrogen provides protective effects on bone density and cardiovascular health.
- **Psychological and Emotional Changes:** Many women experience mood swings, anxiety, and depression during menopause due to hormonal changes. These symptoms can sometimes be severe and may require therapeutic intervention.

Postmenopausal Years (Ages 55 and beyond)

The postmenopausal years follow the end of menstruation and are often associated with a reduction in the risk of pregnancy but an increase in age-related health concerns. Estrogen levels remain low, and women become more susceptible to various chronic health conditions due to the loss of hormonal protection.

- **Health Risks:** After menopause, women are at higher risk for osteoporosis, cardiovascular disease, urinary incontinence, and some cancers, particularly breast and ovarian cancer. Hormonal changes also affect metabolism, leading to potential weight gain and changes in body composition.

- **Mental and Cognitive Health:** Cognitive decline, including memory loss and difficulty concentrating, can become more pronounced in the postmenopausal years. However, many women experience improved mental clarity and emotional stability once the hormonal fluctuations of menopause subside.
- **Sexual Health:** Sexual health and libido may change, often due to vaginal dryness, reduced estrogen, and changes in sexual desire. Many women need to explore new ways to maintain intimacy in their relationships.

1. **Health Considerations for Each Stage**

Each of a woman's four life stages brings its own set of health considerations. Proper care and attention to each stage can help mitigate the risks associated with these changes.

Adolescence

- **Nutrition:** Proper nutrition during adolescence is essential for growth and development. A balanced diet rich in vitamins and minerals, especially calcium and iron, is necessary for developing bones, muscles, and overall health.
- **Mental Health:** Adolescence is a time of emotional upheaval and identity development, and mental health support is crucial. Issues such as depression, anxiety, and eating disorders may surface during this stage.
- **Preventive Healthcare:** This is a key time to establish good habits, such as regular physical activity and good hygiene. Vaccinations, screenings, and discussions about sexual health are essential at this stage.

Reproductive Years

- **Contraception and Family Planning:** Contraception choices can vary based on a woman's health, lifestyle, and reproductive goals. It's essential to consult a healthcare provider to choose the best method for individual needs.
- **Sexual Health:** Regular screenings for sexually transmitted infections (STIs) and cervical cancer (Pap smears) are recommended during these years. Ensuring safe sexual practices is critical.
- **Pregnancy and Postpartum Care:** Regular prenatal checkups are necessary for monitoring fetal development and maternal health during pregnancy. Postpartum care, including physical recovery and mental health screening (for postpartum depression), is equally important.

- **Mental Health and Work-Life Balance:** Many women experience stress balancing career, family, and social obligations. Managing stress through physical activity, social support, and relaxation techniques is vital.

Menopause

- **Hormone Replacement Therapy (HRT):** Hormone replacement therapy may be considered for alleviating the symptoms of menopause, such as hot flashes, night sweats, and mood swings. However, HRT carries risks, such as an increased risk of certain cancers and blood clots, and should be discussed with a healthcare provider.
- **Bone Health:** Postmenopausal women should focus on maintaining bone health through weight-bearing exercises, adequate calcium and vitamin D intake, and medications that help reduce bone loss.
- **Cardiovascular Health:** As estrogen levels decrease, the risk of heart disease increases. Women in this stage should monitor their cholesterol levels and blood pressure and engage in regular cardiovascular exercise to maintain heart health.
- **Mental and Emotional Health:** Dealing with symptoms like mood swings, anxiety, and depression is crucial. Psychological support, therapy, and stress management techniques can aid in coping with the emotional transitions.

Postmenopausal Years

- **Bone and Joint Health:** To prevent osteoporosis and fractures, a continued focus on bone health through weight-bearing exercises, calcium, and vitamin D supplementation is essential.
- **Cancer Screenings:** Regular cancer screenings, including mammograms and pelvic exams, are crucial for detecting any signs of breast or gynecological cancers early.
- **Sexual Health:** Addressing changes in sexual health through the use of lubricants or vaginal estrogen treatments can improve quality of life.

- **Mental Health:** Cognitive health should be a priority in the postmenopausal years, as early interventions can help prevent dementia and cognitive decline. Social engagement and mental exercises help maintain cognitive function.

1. **Transitioning Between Life Stages and Its Impact on Health**

Many women find transitioning from one life stage to the next difficult. The shift in hormone levels, changes in physical appearance, and emotional impact of these transitions require adaptability and self-care.

- **From Adolescence to Reproductive Years:** This transition marks a significant shift in hormonal balance, with the onset of menstruation, ovulation, and sexual maturity. As their bodies adjust, women may experience physical discomforts like menstrual cramps and mood swings. Developing healthy habits during this time sets the foundation for lifelong well-being.

- **From Reproductive Years to Menopause:** The gradual shift toward menopause can be physically and emotionally challenging. Hormonal fluctuations cause symptoms like hot flashes, irregular periods, and mood disturbances. Women may need support in managing these changes and guidance on available medical interventions, such as HRT or natural remedies.

- **From Menopause to Post-Menopause:** The postmenopausal years often feel like a time of renewal, with many women experiencing improved mental clarity and reduced reproductive health worries.

Chapter 3: Physical Health Essentials

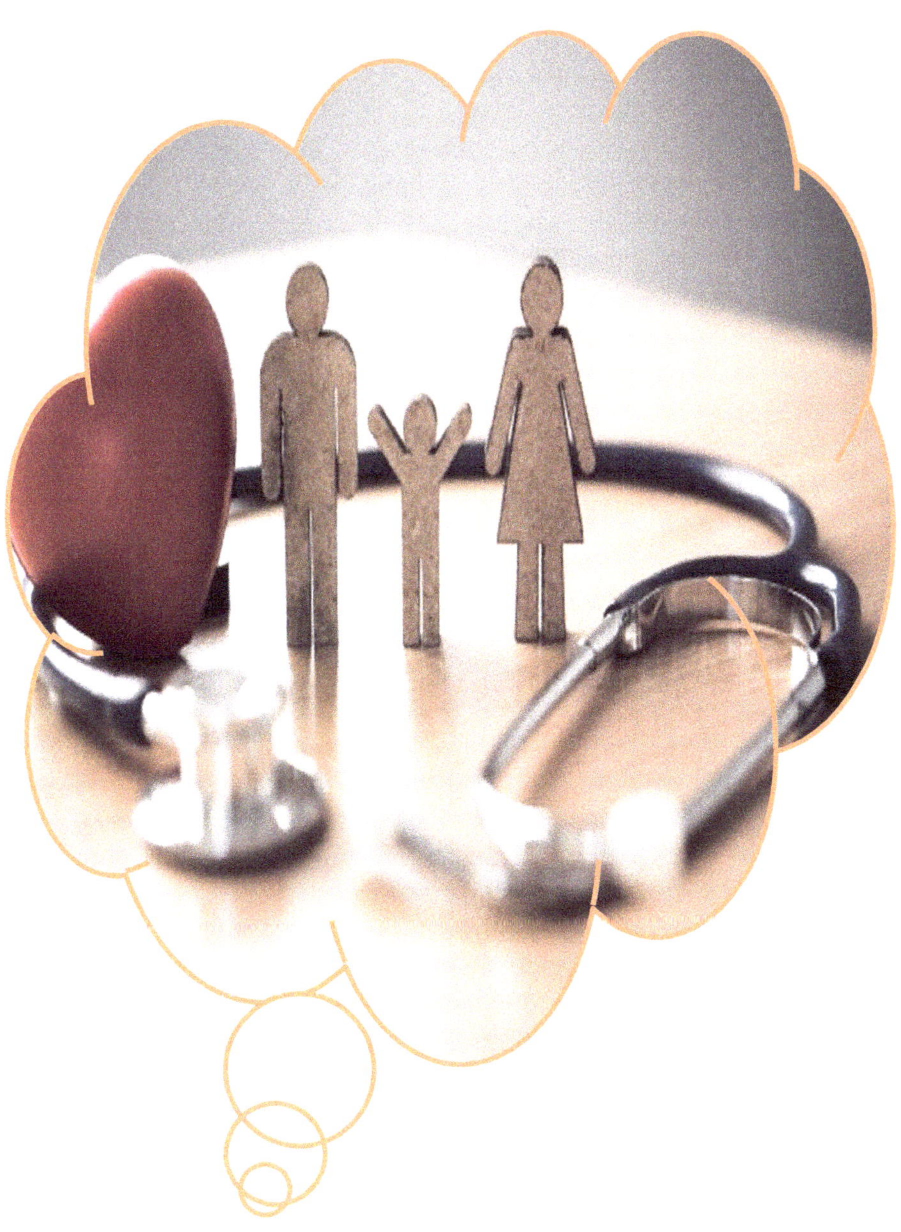

Introduction

Physical health is a crucial aspect of overall well-being, and individuals need to engage in behaviors that promote and maintain their physical health throughout life. For women, this involves regular monitoring, understanding unique health needs, and addressing specific conditions that may arise due to gender-related factors, hormonal changes, and lifestyle choices. This chapter provides an in-depth look into the importance of regular health check-ups and key physical health metrics that are particularly relevant for women and explores chronic conditions prevalent in women's health.

Importance of Regular Check-ups and Screenings

Regular health check-ups and screenings are fundamental to maintaining good health, preventing disease, and identifying health issues early. Preventive health measures are significant for women due to their unique biological and hormonal needs. Here, we will discuss the significance of these screenings and check-ups and the recommended guidelines.

1. **Preventive Care and Early Detection**

Regular check-ups allow healthcare providers to detect health issues before they become serious. Early detection of conditions like cancer, cardiovascular disease, or diabetes can be life-saving. For example, mammograms and Pap smears help in the early detection of breast cancer and cervical cancer, respectively, significantly increasing the chances of successful treatment.

1. **Monitoring Reproductive Health**

Reproductive health is a key aspect of women's overall well-being. Regular gynecological check-ups ensure that any potential issues related to menstruation, fertility, or menopause are addressed promptly. Conditions such as polycystic ovary syndrome (PCOS), endometriosis, or fibroids can be detected early and treated more effectively when regular check-ups are part of a woman's health routine.

1. **Management of Risk Factors**

Regular screenings benefit women with known risk factors for specific health conditions. These screenings help manage conditions like osteoporosis, hypertension, and high cholesterol early on. For instance, women with a family history of breast cancer can undergo genetic testing to assess their risk and adopt preventative strategies. Similarly, routine blood pressure checks can prevent heart disease by catching early signs of hypertension.

1. **Encouraging Healthy Lifestyle Choices**

Routine health assessments also allow healthcare professionals to discuss and recommend healthier lifestyle choices. This may include diet, exercise, smoking cessation, and mental health advice. Women often manage multiple roles, including work, family, and social obligations, so a regular health check-up reminds them to prioritize their health.

1. **Mental and Emotional Well-being**

Physical health is interconnected with mental and emotional well-being. Regular check-ups give women a chance to discuss concerns related to stress, anxiety, depression, and other mental health issues. Many chronic conditions, such as heart disease, are linked to psychological stress, so addressing mental health concerns is a crucial part of maintaining physical health.

Key Physical Health Metrics for Women

Women have unique health needs that require attention to specific physical health metrics. By regularly monitoring these metrics, women can better understand their health status and take preventive measures when necessary. This section explores the essential physical health metrics for women and their significance.

1. **Body Mass Index (BMI)**

BMI is a widely used tool for assessing whether an individual is at a healthy weight for their height. A BMI within the range of 18.5 to 24.9 is considered normal, while anything below is classified as underweight, and above 30 is considered obese. Maintaining a healthy weight is crucial for preventing conditions like type 2 diabetes, heart disease, and joint problems. However, it is essential to note that BMI is not always a perfect measure, as it doesn't consider muscle mass and fat distribution, which can vary across individuals.

1. **Blood Pressure**

Monitoring blood pressure is essential for women, as high blood pressure (hypertension) can lead to heart disease, stroke, kidney failure, and other health issues. The American Heart Association recommends that women have their blood pressure checked at least once every two years. Women should aim to keep their blood pressure below 120/80 mmHg. High blood pressure is often called the "silent killer" because it may not show symptoms but can be damaging over time.

1. **Cholesterol Levels**

Cholesterol plays a vital role in the body, but having high levels of low-density lipoprotein (LDL) cholesterol or total cholesterol can increase the risk of heart disease and stroke. The recommended levels for total cholesterol are under 200 mg/dL. A ratio of HDL to LDL cholesterol is also important, as higher levels of HDL (the "good" cholesterol) are protective against heart disease. Women are often advised to have their cholesterol checked regularly, particularly after the age of 45 or earlier, if they have risk factors for heart disease.

1. **Blood Sugar Levels**

Maintaining normal blood sugar levels is crucial for preventing type 2 diabetes. Women should have their blood sugar levels monitored regularly, especially if they have risk factors such as obesity or a family history of diabetes. Fasting blood glucose levels should be below 100 mg/dL. Women with blood sugar levels between 100 and 125 mg/dL are considered to have prediabetes, while levels above 126 mg/dL indicate diabetes.

1. **Bone Density**

Osteoporosis, a condition that weakens bones and increases fracture risk, is prevalent among postmenopausal women due to a decrease in estrogen levels. A bone density test, typically performed with a dual-energy X-ray absorptiometry (DXA) scan, measures the strength of the bones and is used to diagnose osteoporosis. Women over 65, or those with risk factors, should get a bone density test to assess their bone health.

1. **Cardiovascular Health**

Heart disease is one of the leading causes of death in women. Key metrics for assessing cardiovascular health include cholesterol levels, blood pressure, and heart rate. In addition to these metrics, women should pay attention to other indicators, such as physical activity levels, diet, and stress management, to maintain a healthy heart.

1. **Hormonal Health**

Hormonal health plays a significant role in women's overall health. Key markers such as estrogen, progesterone, and thyroid hormone levels are essential for reproductive health, metabolic function, and emotional well-being. Imbalances in these hormones can lead to conditions like irregular periods, fertility issues, thyroid disorders, and menopause-related symptoms.

1. **Physical Fitness and Activity Levels**

Tracking physical activity levels and maintaining a fitness routine are essential for women's health. Physical fitness is associated with reduced risks of chronic diseases like cardiovascular disease, type 2 diabetes, and certain cancers. Women should aim for at least 150 minutes of moderate-intensity aerobic activity each week and strength training exercises at least two days a week.

Understanding Chronic Conditions Prevalent in Women

Women face a variety of chronic health conditions that are more common or have a more significant impact on them than on men. These conditions may arise from genetic, hormonal, or lifestyle factors. Understanding these chronic conditions is crucial for prevention, early detection, and management.

1. **Heart Disease**

Heart disease is the leading cause of death for women worldwide. Women often experience different symptoms from men, such as shortness of breath, nausea, and fatigue. Risk factors for heart disease include high blood pressure, high cholesterol, smoking, diabetes, and a family history of cardiovascular disease. Women must be aware of these risk factors and take preventive measures, including lifestyle modifications such as exercise, diet, and stress management.

1. **Breast Cancer**

Breast cancer is the most common cancer among women. Early detection through mammograms and self-breast exams is essential for improving survival rates. Women should start regular screenings at age 40 and continue every two years until age 74, depending on risk factors and family history. Women who have a family history of breast cancer or genetic predispositions, such as BRCA gene mutations, should consider more frequent screenings and preventive measures.

1. **Osteoporosis**

As mentioned earlier, osteoporosis is more common in women, particularly postmenopausal women. Decreased estrogen levels contribute to a reduction in bone density, making bones more fragile and prone to fractures. Preventive measures include adequate calcium and vitamin D intake, weight-bearing exercises, and bone density testing.

1. **Diabetes**

Women are at risk of developing both type 1 and type 2 diabetes. Gestational diabetes, which occurs during pregnancy, is also a significant risk factor for developing type 2 diabetes later in life. Managing blood sugar levels through diet, exercise, and medication (if necessary) is crucial for preventing complications associated with diabetes, such as nerve damage, kidney disease, and heart disease.

1. **Autoimmune Diseases**

Women are more likely than men to develop autoimmune diseases, such as lupus, rheumatoid arthritis, and multiple sclerosis. In these diseases, the body's immune system mistakenly attacks healthy cells and tissues. Symptoms vary widely depending on the disease but may include joint pain, fatigue, and organ dysfunction. Early diagnosis and treatment are essential to managing these conditions and improving quality of life.

1. **Depression and Anxiety**

Mental health conditions like depression and anxiety are prevalent among women, often linked to hormonal fluctuations, societal pressures, and caregiving responsibilities. These conditions can also have physical health implications, such as contributing to chronic pain, digestive issues, and cardiovascular disease. Women should seek professional help if they experience symptoms of depression or anxiety.

1. **Polycystic Ovary Syndrome (PCOS)**

PCOS is a common hormonal disorder affecting women of reproductive age. It can cause irregular periods, infertility, and excess androgen production, leading to symptoms such as acne and excess hair growth. PCOS is also associated with an increased

Chapter 4: Mental Well-Being

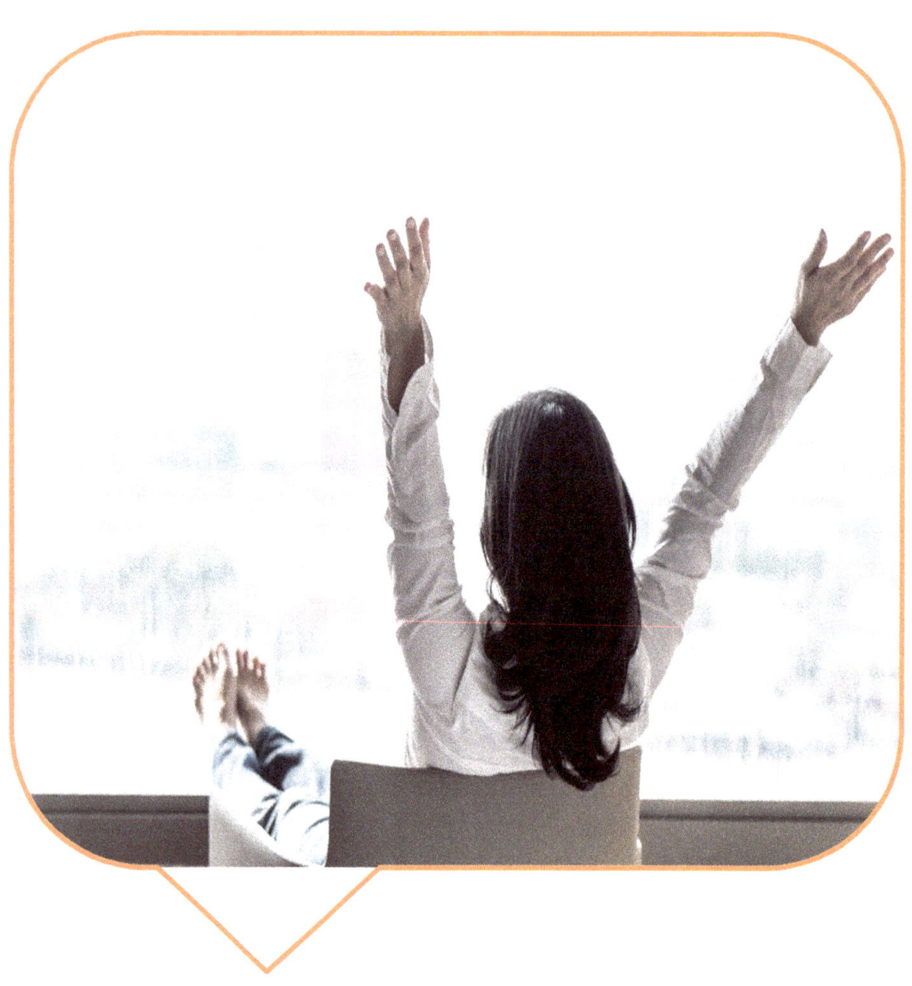

Introduction

Mental well-being is integral to overall health, influencing how individuals think, feel, and act. The connection between psychological and physical health is profound, as mental states affect bodily functions and vice versa. In particular, women often experience unique mental health challenges that are influenced by a variety of factors, including hormonal changes, societal pressures, and personal life events. This chapter explores the intricate relationship between mental and physical health, highlights common mental health issues women face, and discusses practical strategies to maintain and improve mental wellness.

1. **The Connection Between Mental and Physical Health**

The relationship between mental and physical health is bidirectional, meaning that each can influence the other. The mind and body are not separate entities but interconnected systems. Mental health issues can lead to physical ailments, and physical health issues can, in turn, exacerbate mental health problems.

Impact of Mental Health on Physical Health

Mental health problems such as anxiety, depression, and chronic stress can manifest in various physical symptoms. Some of the most common physical symptoms include:

- **Immune System Suppression**: Chronic stress and depression can weaken the immune system, making individuals more susceptible to infections.
- **Heart Disease**: Long-term mental health problems, particularly stress, have been linked to increased risk of heart disease and high blood pressure.
- **Chronic Pain**: Mental health disorders can amplify the perception of physical pain. Conditions like fibromyalgia or chronic headaches may be worsened by stress or depression.
- **Sleep Disorders**: Anxiety and depression are frequently associated with sleep disturbances, which can, in turn, negatively impact physical health by leading to fatigue, impaired immune function, and cognitive decline.
- **Gastrointestinal Issues**: Mental health issues are often associated with gastrointestinal disturbances, such as irritable bowel syndrome (IBS), stomach ulcers, and indigestion.

Impact of Physical Health on Mental Health

On the other hand, chronic physical health conditions can also lead to mental health issues. For example:

- **Chronic Illness**: Living with chronic conditions like diabetes, cancer, or arthritis can lead to feelings of helplessness, anxiety, and depression.

- **Physical Disabilities**: Injuries or disabilities that affect mobility or independence may contribute to isolation, stress, and anxiety.
- **Hormonal Imbalances**: Changes in hormone levels, particularly in women (e.g., menopause or pregnancy), can cause mood swings, depression, and anxiety.

Understanding this connection makes it clear that physical and mental health must be addressed in an integrated manner to ensure overall well-being. Effective treatment and prevention strategies should consider both the mind and body, emphasizing the importance of a holistic approach to health.

1. **Common Mental Health Issues in Women**

While mental health problems affect both men and women, women are statistically more likely to experience certain mental health conditions, often due to hormonal, biological, and social factors. Among the most common mental health issues affecting women are anxiety, depression, and eating disorders. Below is a detailed examination of these conditions:

Anxiety Disorders

Anxiety is characterized by excessive worry, fear, and nervousness, often without a clear cause. Anxiety disorders are the most common mental health issues women face, with women being twice as likely to be diagnosed as men.

- **Generalized Anxiety Disorder (GAD)**: Women with GAD often experience constant worry about various aspects of life, including work, health, and relationships. This constant worry can lead to fatigue, irritability, and physical symptoms like muscle tension and sleep problems.
- **Panic Disorder**: Panic disorder is marked by sudden and intense feelings of fear or dread, often accompanied by physical symptoms such as heart palpitations, sweating, dizziness, and shortness of breath.
- **Post-Traumatic Stress Disorder (PTSD)**: Women are more likely to develop PTSD, particularly following traumatic events such as sexual assault or domestic violence. Flashbacks, nightmares, and an overwhelming sense of fear or dread characterize PTSD.
- **Social Anxiety Disorder**: This type of anxiety is characterized by extreme fear of being judged or embarrassed in social situations, leading to avoidance of social interactions and isolation.

Causes and Risk Factors for Anxiety in Women

The causes of anxiety are complex and often involve a combination of genetic, environmental, and psychological factors. Women may be more vulnerable to anxiety due to:

- **Hormonal Changes**: Pregnancy, menstruation, and menopause can cause significant hormonal fluctuations, which may contribute to anxiety.

- **Trauma and Abuse**: Women are more likely to experience trauma and abuse, both of which can trigger anxiety disorders.
- **Social Pressures**: Women often face societal pressures to meet high standards in various roles (e.g., as caregivers, professionals, and family members), which can contribute to stress and anxiety.

Depression

Depression is a mood disorder characterized by persistent sadness, loss of interest or pleasure in activities, and feelings of hopelessness. Women are nearly twice as likely to experience depression as men.

- **Major Depressive Disorder (MDD)**: This is the most severe form of depression, often resulting in significant impairment in daily functioning. Symptoms include deep sadness, fatigue, trouble concentrating, and thoughts of suicide.
- **Persistent Depressive Disorder (PDD)**: Also known as dysthymia, PDD is a chronic form of depression lasting for at least two years. While not as severe as MDD, PDD can still interfere with daily life and cause significant distress.
- **Postpartum Depression**: Many women experience depressive symptoms following childbirth, a condition that is more severe than the "baby blues" commonly encountered in the weeks after delivery.

Causes and Risk Factors for Depression in Women

Depression in women can be triggered or worsened by:

- **Hormonal Changes**: Fluctuations in hormones, particularly estrogen and progesterone, can contribute to mood changes and increase the risk of depression.
- **Genetic Factors**: A family history of depression can increase the likelihood of developing the condition.
- **Life Stressors**: Women may experience unique life stressors such as caregiving responsibilities, work-life balance challenges, and societal expectations, all of which can increase vulnerability to depression.
- **Trauma and Abuse**: Like anxiety, depression can result from past trauma, particularly experiences of abuse or loss.

Eating Disorders

Eating disorders such as anorexia nervosa, bulimia nervosa, and binge-eating disorder are more prevalent in women. These disorders are often linked to negative body image and a desire for control over one's life or environment.

- **Anorexia Nervosa**: Characterized by an extreme fear of gaining weight, anorexia involves self-imposed starvation and excessive weight loss.
- **Bulimia Nervosa**: This involves cycles of binge eating followed by compensatory behaviors such as vomiting or excessive exercise to avoid weight gain.

- **Binge-eating disorder** is characterized by recurring episodes of eating large quantities of food in a short period, often accompanied by feelings of shame or guilt.

Causes and Risk Factors for Eating Disorders in Women

- **Cultural Pressures**: Western ideals of beauty often promote thinness, which can contribute to body dissatisfaction and disordered eating behaviors.
- **Psychological Factors**: Many women with eating disorders have underlying issues related to control, perfectionism, or a history of trauma.
- **Biological Factors**: Genetic predispositions and brain chemistry may play a role in the development of eating disorders.

1. **Strategies for Maintaining Mental Wellness**

Maintaining mental wellness requires proactive and reactive strategies focusing on emotional, psychological, and social well-being. It involves building resilience, managing stress, and seeking help when necessary. Below are several key strategies for maintaining mental wellness:

Self-Care Practices

Self-care involves intentional activities that promote physical, emotional, and mental health. Some effective self-care practices include:

- **Physical Exercise**: Regular physical activity releases endorphins known to improve mood and reduce anxiety. Exercise also helps with sleep, boosts self-esteem, and provides social connection opportunities.
- **Adequate Sleep**: Good sleep hygiene, including maintaining a regular sleep schedule and creating a restful sleep environment, is essential for mental wellness.
- **Balanced Diet**: A well-rounded diet with plenty of fruits, vegetables, whole grains, and lean proteins can support brain health and improve mood regulation.

- **Relaxation Techniques**: Practices like yoga, deep breathing exercises, progressive muscle relaxation, and mindfulness meditation can reduce stress and improve overall mental health.

Social Support

Strong social connections are essential for maintaining mental health. Building and nurturing relationships with family, friends, and community members provides emotional support, reduces feelings of isolation, and fosters a sense of belonging. Women, in particular, tend to thrive with a solid support network.

- **Therapy and Counseling**: Seeking professional help when needed is crucial in maintaining mental wellness. Therapists or counselors can provide tools to manage mental health conditions, such as anxiety or depression, and help individuals navigate life's challenges.
- **Support Groups**: Participating in support groups for women facing similar mental health challenges can provide a sense of understanding and solidarity.

Stress Management

Managing stress effectively is vital for preventing burnout and improving mental resilience. Strategies for managing stress include:

- **Time Management**: Prioritizing tasks and setting realistic goals can prevent overwhelming feelings.
- **Mindfulness**: Practicing mindfulness involves staying present in the moment and can reduce stress and anxiety.
- **Journaling**: Writing down thoughts and feelings can help process emotions and reduce stress.

Seeking Professional Help

When self-care strategies are insufficient, seeking help from a mental health professional is essential. Therapy modalities such as Cognitive Behavioral

Chapter 5: Reproductive Health

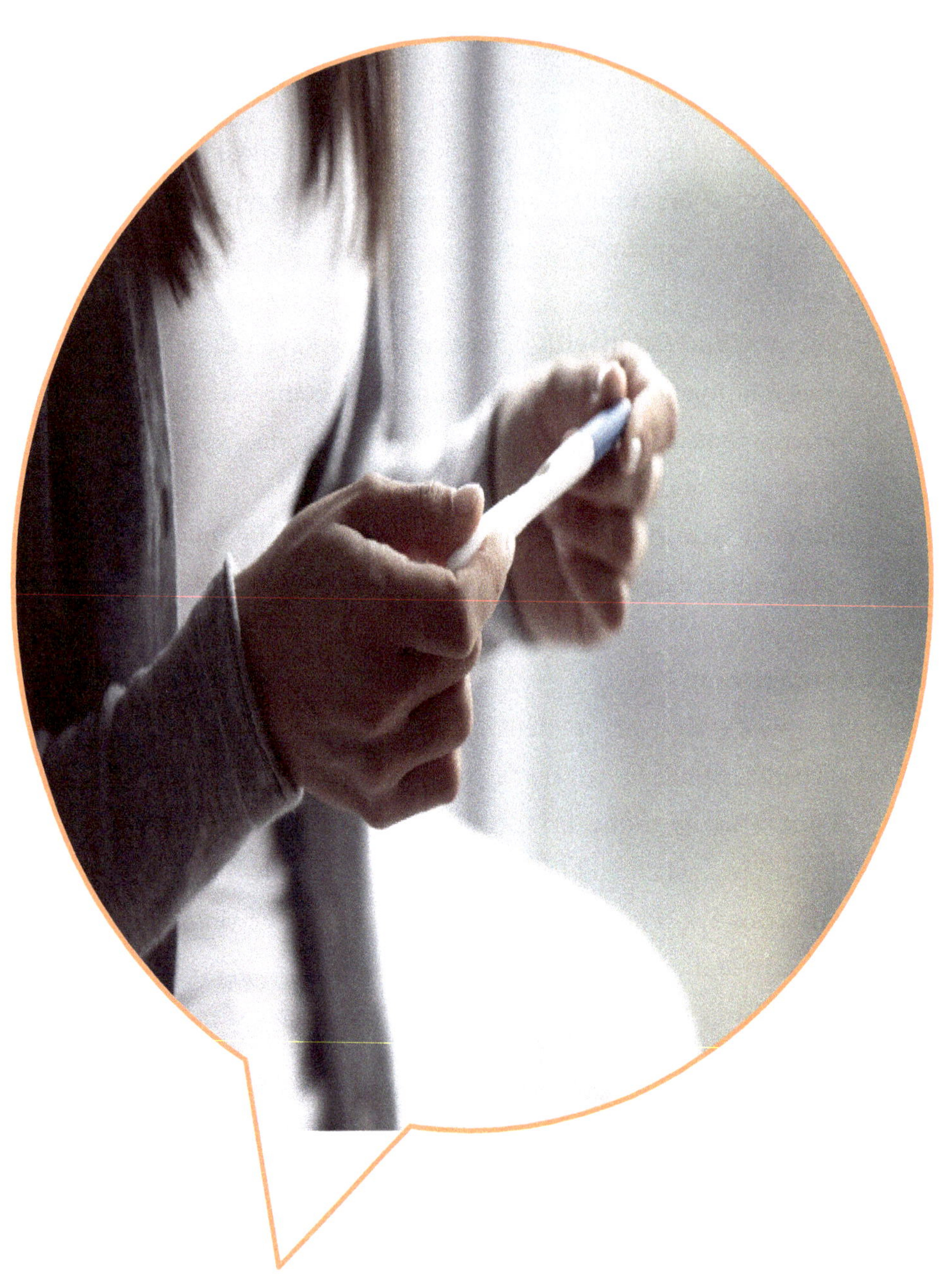

Reproductive health refers to the state of physical, mental, and social well-being in all matters related to the reproductive system, including the processes of reproduction, sexual health, and the ability to enjoy a satisfying and safe sexual life without discrimination or violence. It encompasses many factors, such as menstruation, fertility, family planning, sexual health, and maternal care, and is critical for overall well-being. Reproductive health is significant not only because it influences individual health outcomes but also because it plays a key role in broader public health issues and societal well-being.

1. **Overview of Reproductive Health and Its Significance**

Reproductive health is essential for the health and well-being of individuals, communities, and populations. It ensures that people can have children if and when they choose and that they can have access to healthcare services and information that prevent reproductive health issues. It also involves quality maternal and neonatal care, access to safe childbirth practices, and a supportive environment for raising healthy children.

Key Aspects of Reproductive Health:

- **Maternal Health**: This includes pregnancy, childbirth, and postpartum care. Good reproductive health practices ensure healthy pregnancies, reduce maternal mortality rates, and provide care during the postnatal period.
- **Sexual Health**: This focuses on the individual's ability to experience sexual satisfaction and well-being. It includes the prevention of sexually transmitted infections (STIs) and sexual violence and ensuring healthy sexual relationships.
- **Fertility and Conception**: The ability to conceive a child and treat infertility. This aspect involves reproductive health education, fertility treatments, and emotional support for individuals facing fertility challenges.

Significance of Reproductive Health:

- **Health Implications**: Poor reproductive health can lead to complications such as infertility, STIs, and maternal and neonatal deaths.
- **Gender Equality**: Addressing reproductive health is crucial for achieving gender equality as it empowers individuals, particularly women, to make informed decisions about their reproductive rights.
- **Economic Development**: Healthy reproductive health policies are linked to improved productivity, better health outcomes for families, and reduced financial burdens on healthcare systems.
- **Societal Impact**: Reproductive health services reduce healthcare costs, promote safe family planning, and allow for the responsible planning of families, leading to sustainable population growth.

1. **Menstrual Health and Menstrual Disorders**

Menstrual health refers to the overall health of the menstrual cycle and the absence of disorders that may interfere with its normal functioning. The menstrual cycle plays a fundamental role in the reproductive system and affects a woman's physical and emotional well-being. It is a complex physiological process influenced by hormonal regulation, and its irregularities can significantly impact women's health.

Menstrual Health:

- **Normal Menstrual Cycle**: The menstrual cycle typically lasts 28 days, although cycles ranging from 21 to 35 days are also standard. When pregnancy does not occur, the uterine lining sheds, which is marked by menstruation. The average length of menstruation is between 3 and 7 days, and blood loss is usually 30-80 milliliters per cycle.
- **Factors Affecting Menstrual Health**: Factors such as nutrition, physical activity, stress levels, and underlying health conditions can affect menstrual health. Hormonal imbalances, lifestyle factors, or genetics can lead to abnormalities in the menstrual cycle.

Menstrual Disorders: Menstrual disorders are common conditions affecting women of reproductive age. These disorders can be indicative of other underlying health problems and often require medical intervention.

1. **Amenorrhea**: The absence of menstruation. Primary amenorrhea refers to the lack of menstruation by age 16, and secondary amenorrhea refers to the absence of periods for 3 or more months after a woman has previously menstruated. Causes include hormonal imbalances, excessive physical activity, stress, or disorders such as polycystic ovary syndrome (PCOS).
2. **Dysmenorrhea**: Painful menstruation. This can be primary (pain without an underlying medical condition) or secondary (pain due to conditions like endometriosis, fibroids, or pelvic inflammatory disease). Pain can be severe and debilitating, affecting a woman's ability to perform daily activities.
3. **Menorrhagia**: Heavy menstrual bleeding, which can lead to anemia and other complications. Fibroids, endometriosis, or other reproductive system conditions may cause it. Heavy bleeding is defined as losing more than 80 milliliters of blood per cycle, often accompanied by prolonged menstruation.
4. **Oligomenorrhea**: Infrequent menstruation, typically defined as cycles longer than 35 days. This condition can be a symptom of polycystic ovary syndrome, thyroid issues, or excessive exercise.
5. **Premenstrual Syndrome (PMS)**: PMS includes physical, emotional, and psychological symptoms occurring in the luteal phase of the

menstrual cycle. Symptoms include mood swings, irritability, fatigue, and bloating. Severe PMS, called premenstrual dysphoric disorder (PMDD), can significantly impact quality of life.

6. **Endometriosis**: A condition in which tissue similar to the lining of the uterus grows outside of the uterus, causing chronic pain, heavy menstrual bleeding, and fertility issues.

Management and Treatment of Menstrual Disorders:

- **Medication**: Pain relievers (e.g., NSAIDs), hormonal treatments (e.g., birth control pills, IUDs), and antifibrinolytics (e.g., tranexamic acid) to reduce bleeding.
- **Lifestyle Changes**: Stress reduction, exercise, a balanced diet, and proper sleep hygiene can help improve menstrual health.
- **Surgical Interventions**: In severe disorders like fibroids or endometriosis, surgery may be required to remove abnormal growths or repair anatomical issues.
- **Alternative Therapies**: Acupuncture, herbal treatments, and physical therapy may provide relief for some women.

1. **Family Planning and Fertility Awareness**

Family planning refers to the conscious decision made by individuals or couples to determine the number and timing of children, often through the use of contraceptive methods and fertility awareness. This aspect of reproductive health is crucial for ensuring that individuals can achieve their desired family size and spacing of children, as well as promote healthier pregnancies and reduce unplanned pregnancies.

Methods of Family Planning:

- **Contraceptive Methods**: There are several types of contraception available for individuals who want to prevent pregnancy.
    - **Hormonal Contraception**: Birth control pills, patches, injections, and intrauterine devices (IUDs) that release hormones like estrogen and progestin to prevent ovulation.
    - **Barrier Methods**: Condoms (male and female), diaphragms, and cervical caps work by physically blocking sperm from reaching the egg.
    - **Permanent Contraception**: Sterilization methods such as vasectomy and tubal ligation provide long-term, irreversible contraception.
    - **Natural Family Planning**: This includes methods like the calendar method, cervical mucus method, and basal body temperature method, which rely on understanding the menstrual cycle to predict fertile days.
- **Fertility Awareness**: This involves tracking signs and symptoms of fertility throughout the menstrual cycle to determine when an individual is most fertile. Key aspects of fertility awareness include:

- **Basal Body Temperature (BBT)**: A slight increase in body temperature after ovulation.
- **Cervical Mucus Monitoring**: The texture and amount of cervical mucus changes throughout the cycle, becoming more transparent and slippery around ovulation.
- **Ovulation Predictor Kits**: These kits detect the luteinizing hormone (LH) surge that occurs just before ovulation.
- **Menstrual Cycle Tracking**: Using apps or calendars to track cycle length and predict ovulation.

Benefits of Family Planning and Fertility Awareness:

- **Empowerment**: Family planning allows individuals to make informed choices about their reproductive health, enabling them to achieve their desired family size and timing.
- **Health Benefits**: Proper family planning reduces the risks associated with unplanned pregnancies, such as maternal health complications, preterm birth, and low birth weight.
- **Economic and Social Benefits**: Effective family planning can contribute to financial stability, educational attainment, and improved quality of life for families. It also promotes gender equality by enabling women to participate in the workforce and education.

Challenges to Family Planning and Fertility Awareness:

- **Access to Contraceptive Methods**: In many regions, access to contraceptives is limited due to factors like cost, lack of availability, or cultural beliefs.
- **Cultural and Religious Barriers**: Family planning and contraception may be discouraged in certain cultures or religious contexts, limiting their widespread use.
- **Knowledge Gaps**: A lack of education and awareness about fertility and reproductive health often leads to misconceptions and improper use of contraceptive methods.
- **Health Risks**: Certain contraceptive methods may have side effects or health risks, which should be managed with medical guidance.

Conclusion:

Reproductive health is essential to overall well-being, encompassing menstrual health, fertility, and family planning. By ensuring access to information and healthcare services, individuals can make informed choices regarding their reproductive health. Though common, menstrual disorders and fertility challenges are treatable with proper care, while family planning empowers individuals to make choices about their reproductive futures. By promoting education, access to healthcare, and the right to make informed decisions, society can ensure that everyone can experience healthy reproductive lives.

Chapter 6: Nutrition for Women

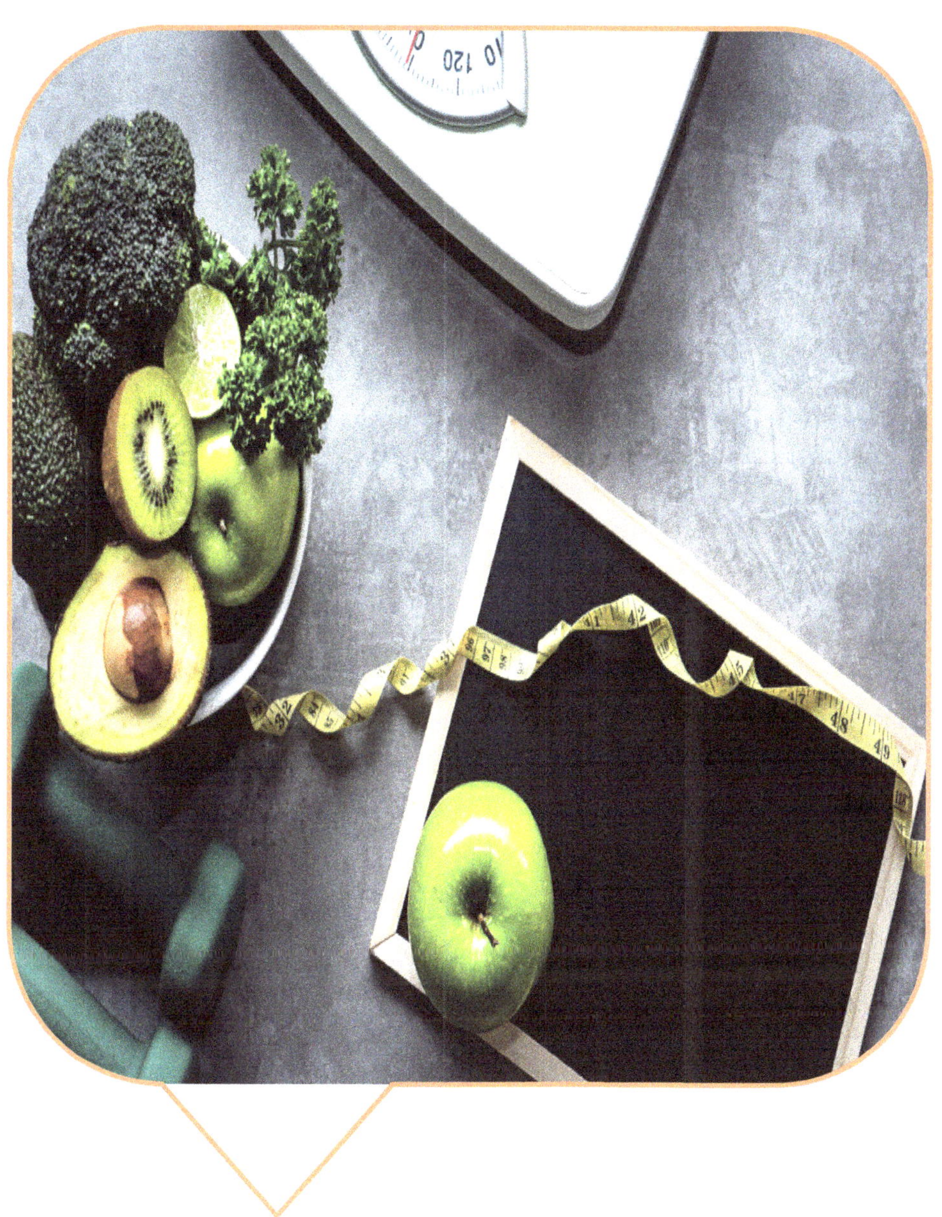

Introduction

Women's nutrition plays a critical role in their overall health and well-being. Due to biological differences and life stage transitions, women's nutritional needs evolve throughout their lifetime. This chapter focuses on understanding these needs and highlights the importance of balanced diets, hydration, and dispelling common myths that can influence dietary choices.

1. **Nutritional Needs at Different Life Stages**

Women's nutritional requirements fluctuate across life stages, including adolescence, pregnancy, lactation, adulthood, and menopause. Each stage involves distinct physiological changes that necessitate tailored nutritional support.

Adolescence (Ages 12-18)

Women's presence is a period of rapid physical and hormonal changes, requiring adequate nutrition to support growth and development. Key considerations for adolescent girls include:

- **Energy Needs**: Adolescents experience growth spurts, increasing their calorie requirements. Adequate energy intake is essential for promoting healthy bone development, muscle mass, and general well-being.
- **Iron**: As menstruation begins, iron needs to increase due to blood loss during periods. Iron-rich foods such as leafy greens, red meat, legumes, and fortified cereals are crucial to avoid iron deficiency anemia.
- **Calcium and Vitamin D**: Bone mass is developed during adolescence, so adequate calcium intake is vital for bone density. Vitamin D is also necessary for calcium absorption. Dairy products, fortified plant-based milk, and exposure to sunlight help meet these needs.
- **Folate**: Folate is essential for preventing neural tube defects in the event of pregnancy, making it a necessary nutrient during adolescence.

Reproductive Years (Ages 19-40)

During these years, a woman's body requires nutritional support for fertility, pregnancy (if applicable), and overall health.

- **Iron**: Ongoing menstruation heightens the need for iron. Low iron levels can lead to fatigue and decreased immune function.
- **Folic Acid**: Essential before and during pregnancy to support healthy fetal development.
- **Protein and Healthy Fats**: These macronutrients are essential for cellular health, hormone production, and reproductive function.
- **Calcium and Vitamin D**: To maintain bone health and avoid the risk of osteoporosis later in life.

Pregnancy and Lactation

Pregnancy and lactation significantly change nutrient needs to support the mother's health and the developing child.

- **Energy and Caloric Intake**: During the second and third trimesters, pregnant women need about 300 extra calories per day, and lactating women require an additional 500 calories per day.
- **Folic Acid and Iron**: Folic acid is crucial during pregnancy for the prevention of birth defects, while iron helps the mother support increased blood volume and prevent anemia.
- **Calcium and Vitamin D**: Increased calcium intake is essential for fetal bone development and to preserve the mother's bone health. Vitamin D supports calcium absorption.
- **Omega-3 Fatty Acids**: These healthy fats are crucial for developing the baby's brain and eyes. Sources include fatty fish like salmon, walnuts, and flaxseeds.

Adulthood (Ages 40-60)

As women enter their 40s and 50s, hormonal changes begin, notably the transition toward menopause.

- **Calcium and Vitamin D**: Bone density begins to decrease as estrogen levels drop. Adequate calcium and vitamin D are even more critical to preventing osteoporosis.
- **Iron**: Iron needs to decrease as menstruation stops. However, maintaining adequate iron levels is still essential for energy and immune function.
- **Protein**: Protein intake helps maintain lean muscle mass, which tends to decrease with age.
- **Healthy Fats**: Heart health becomes a priority, and omega-3 fatty acids, found in fatty fish, walnuts, and flaxseeds, are essential for cardiovascular health.

Post menopause (Ages 60+)

Menopause marks the end of a woman's reproductive years and introduces changes that necessitate further adjustments to nutrition.

- **Calcium and Vitamin D**: Due to decreased bone mass, postmenopausal women are at increased risk of osteoporosis and fractures. Calcium, vitamin D, and weight-bearing exercises are essential.
- **Protein**: Maintaining muscle mass becomes crucial to overall strength and mobility. Protein-rich foods such as lean meats, legumes, and dairy are vital.
- **Heart Health**: The risk of cardiovascular disease increases after menopause, making a heart-healthy diet rich in women's and low in saturated fats a priority.

- **Hydration**: Dehydration can become more common in older women, making adequate fluid intake even more important.

1. **Importance of a Balanced Diet and Hydration**

Balanced Diet

A balanced diet provides the nutrients the body needs to function optimally. A variety of foods, including fruits, vegetables, whole grains, protein sources, and healthy fats, are essential for maintaining good health.

- **Macronutrients**:
  - **Carbohydrates**: Provide energy and help maintain blood sugar levels. Whole grains, fruits, and vegetables are excellent sources of complex carbohydrates, which are rich in fiber and essential for digestive health.
  - **Proteins** are crucial for muscle repair, immune function, and hormone regulation. Lean meats, beans, nuts, and legumes are excellent sources.
  - **Fats**: Healthy fats, such as omega-3 fatty acids, are necessary for brain function, heart health, and hormone production. Sources include avocados, nuts, seeds, and fatty fish.
- **Micronutrients**:
  - **Vitamins** A, C, D, E, and B-complex vitamins are critical for immune function, skin health, bone density, and energy production.
  - **Minerals**: Calcium, iron, magnesium, and zinc play vital roles in bone health, oxygen transport, and cellular function.

Hydration

Water is crucial for every bodily function, including digestion, nutrient absorption, temperature regulation, and waste elimination. A woman's water needs vary based on age, activity level, and environment.

- **General Guidelines**: Women should aim to drink at least 2.7 liters (91 ounces) of water daily, but this amount can vary. Pregnant or breastfeeding women may require more fluids.
- **Signs of Dehydration** include dry skin, fatigue, headaches, and dark yellow urine. Alzheimer's disease also shows signs of dehydration. Ensuring adequate fluid intake is essential, especially during physical activity or in hot climates.

1. **Common Dietary Myths and Misconceptions**

Numerous myths surround women's diets, often leading to confusion or unhealthy dietary habits. Understanding these misconceptions is essential for making informed, science-backed decisions.

Myth 1: Carbs Are Bad for You

Carbohydrates are often demonized in fad diets, but they are essential to a balanced diet. The key is choosing complex carbohydrates, which are high in fiber and take longer to digest, providing sustained energy. Whole grains, vegetables, and legumes are excellent sources of healthy carbs.

Myth 2: Eating Fat Will Make You Fat

Not all fats are created equal. Healthy fats, such as monounsaturated and polyunsaturated fats, support heart health, brain function, and hormone balance. The focus should be on limiting trans fats and saturated fats found in processed and fried foods. Healthy fat sources include avocados, nuts, seeds, and olive oil.

Myth 3: Low-Calorie Diets Are Always Effective

While reducing caloric intake can help with weight loss, highly low-calorie diets are unsustainable and can lead to nutrient deficiencies, muscle loss, and metabolic slowdown. Instead of drastically cutting calories, focus on portion control, balanced meals, and regular physical activity for long-term health and weight management.

Myth 4: Soy Causes Hormonal Imbalance

Soy contains phytoestrogens, plant compounds that mimic estrogen in the body. Some fear that consuming soy may lead to hormonal imbalance, but research shows moderate soy consumption is safe for most women. Soy can provide essential nutrients like protein, fiber, and healthy fats.

Myth 5: Detox Diets Are Necessary for Good Health

The idea of "detoxing" through juices or restrictive diets is popular but unfounded. The body naturally detoxifies itself through organs like the liver and kidneys. Focusing on a well-rounded, nutrient-dense diet is far more effective for long-term health than attempting to detox with extreme diets.

Myth 6: You Need to Skip Meals to Lose Weight

Skipping meals can lead to overeating later and may negatively affect metabolism. Regular Balan women's and snacks throughout the day help maintain energy levels, support muscle mass, and prevent overeating.

Conclusion

Nutritional needs for women vary across different life stages, from adolescence to post menopause. A balanced diet rich in essential nutrients and adequate hydration are key to maintaining health and preventing chronic diseases. By dispelling common dietary myths and focusing on evidence-based nutrition, women can empower themselves to make healthy food choices and enjoy a better quality of life.

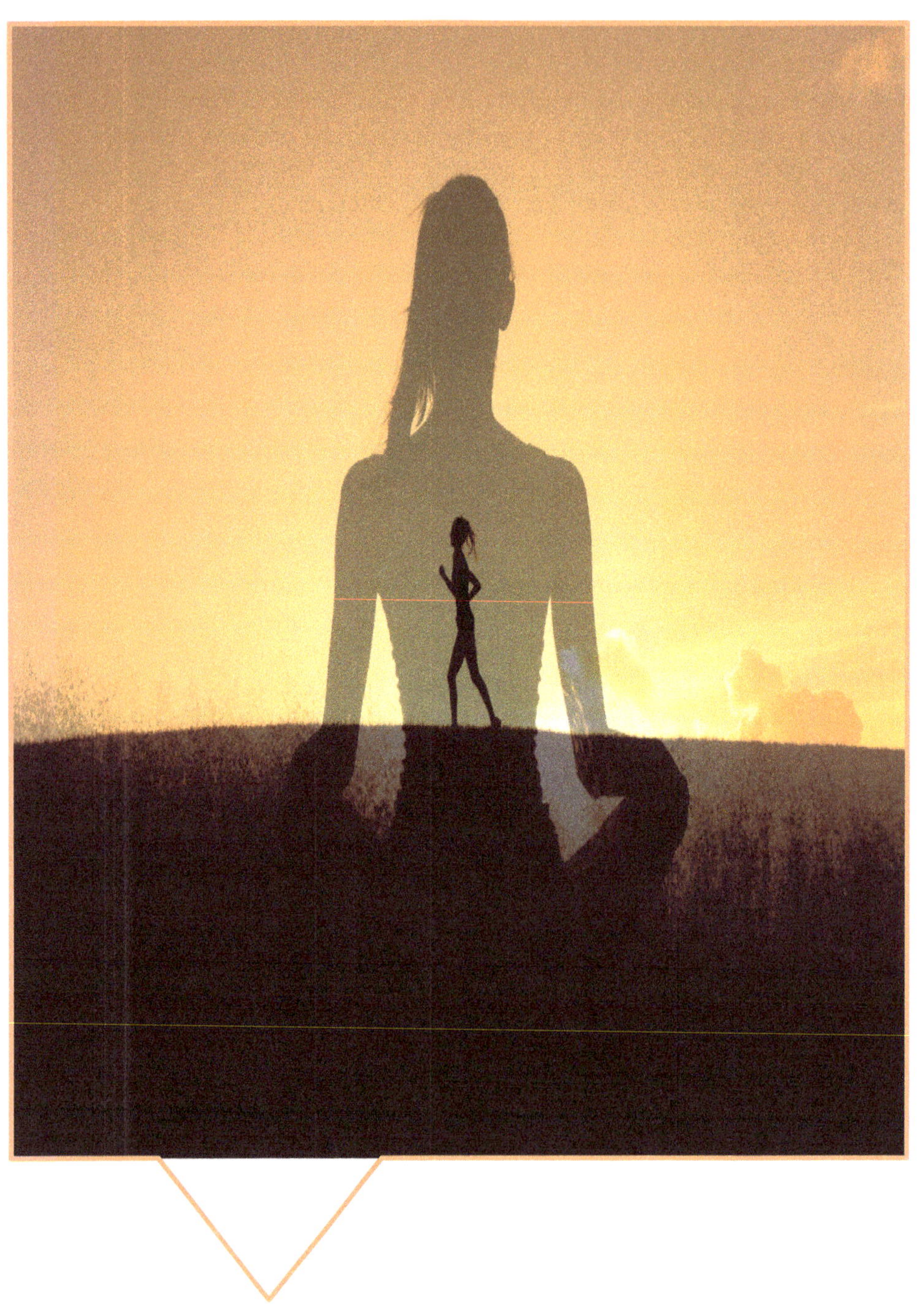

1. Introduction to Exercise and Physical Activity for Women

Physical activity, encompassing exercise and daily movement, is crucial for maintaining and improving health. For women, regular exercise is vital for physical fitness and contributes significantly to emotional well-being and overall quality of life. From adolescence through menopause and beyond, women's bodies undergo various changes that can impact physical activity needs, abilities, and preferences. This chapter explores the benefits of regular exercise for women, identifies exercises suitable for different life stages, and provides strategies for creating a sustainable fitness routine.

1. Benefits of Regular Exercise for Women

2.1 Physical Health Benefits

Cardiovascular Health

Regular exercise strengthens the heart, improves circulation, and lowers blood pressure. It reduces the risk of cardiovascular diseases (CVD) such as heart disease, stroke, and high cholesterol, which are common concerns among women as they age. Cardiovascular fitness is also linked to better lung capacity, which contributes to overall health.

Musculoskeletal Strength

As women age, they become more susceptible to osteoporosis and muscle loss (sarcopenia). Exercise, particularly weight-bearing and resistance activities, helps maintain bone density and muscle strength. This reduces the risk of falls and fractures, which are more common in older women.

Metabolic Health

Exercise is crucial in managing weight, reducing body fat, and increasing lean muscle mass. This, in turn, helps prevent obesity, type 2 diabetes, and metabolic syndrome. Weight management through exercise also improves insulin sensitivity, which helps prevent and manage diabetes.

Improved Flexibility and Mobility

Regular exercise, especially stretching and yoga, improves flexibility and joint mobility. This is particularly important for women, who may experience joint stiffness and loss of range of motion as they age, often exacerbated by hormonal changes such as those associated with menopause.

Boosted Immune System

Moderate exercise enhances immune function, making it easier to fight off infections. It can also reduce the risk of chronic diseases, such as autoimmune conditions, by promoting overall physical health.

2.2 Mental and Emotional Health Benefits

Reduced Stress and Anxiety

Exercise has been shown to reduce cortisol (the stress hormone) levels in the body. It also stimulates the production of endorphins, which are natural mood lifters. As a result, regular physical activity can reduce stress, anxiety, and depression, conditions that many women face, particularly during times of hormonal fluctuation such as pregnancy or menopause.

Enhanced Cognitive Function

Exercise has been linked to improved cognitive function and a reduced risk of cognitive decline. Women are at a higher risk of dementia and Alzheimer's disease as they age. Regular physical activity can improve memory, focus, and overall brain health, potentially delaying the onset of cognitive decline.

Improved Sleep

Engaging in physical activity can improve sleep quality. Women often experience sleep disturbances due to hormonal changes, pregnancy, or menopause. Regular exercise helps regulate circadian rhythms and promotes more restful sleep.

2.3 Long-term Health Benefits

Reduced Risk of Chronic Diseases

Exercise has a protective effect against chronic conditions such as type 2 diabetes, high blood pressure, arthritis, and certain types of cancer (e.g., breast and colon cancer). Regular physical activity also helps maintain the health of vital organs like the liver, kidneys, and lungs.

Increased Longevity

Engaging in regular physical activity has been shown to increase life expectancy. Women who exercise consistently live longer and are less likely to suffer from debilitating diseases in their later years.

Better Quality of Life in Later Years

As women age, maintaining mobility, strength, and mental clarity is crucial. Regular exercise improves quality of life by helping women stay independent for longer and reducing the risks associated with falls, fractures, and other age-related issues.

1. Types of Exercises Suitable for Different Life Stages

3.1 Exercise During Adolescence (12-18 Years)

Key Considerations:

- Bone health is essential during this stage, as bone mass is still developing.
- Hormonal fluctuations during puberty may affect energy levels and mood.

Recommended Exercises:

- **Aerobic Exercise**: Activities like swimming, running, cycling, and dancing help improve cardiovascular health.
- **Strength Training**: Light to moderate resistance training using body weight (e.g., push-ups, squats) or resistance bands can enhance muscle strength and bone density.

- **Sports Participation**: Involvement in team sports (basketball, soccer, volleyball) promotes social interaction and cardiovascular fitness.
- **Flexibility Exercises**: Stretching or yoga can improve flexibility and reduce the risk of injury.

3.2 Exercise During Young Adulthood (19-35 Years)

Key Considerations:

- This is a period of peak physical fitness, but women may experience changes due to pregnancy and childbirth.
- It's a crucial time for maintaining metabolic health.

Recommended Exercises:

- **Cardiovascular Exercise**: Running, cycling, or swimming are excellent ways to maintain heart health and improve stamina.
- **Strength Training**: Weightlifting or resistance exercises help maintain muscle mass, which naturally declines as women age.
- **Flexibility and Mobility Work**: Yoga, Pilates, or dynamic stretching improves flexibility, reduces stress, and supports joint health.
- **Core Strengthening**: Exercises focusing on the core, such as planks or Pilates, can support spinal health, especially post-pregnancy.

Considerations for Pregnancy and Postpartum:

Moderate exercises such as walking, swimming, and prenatal yoga are ideal during pregnancy. Postpartum, women can gradually reintroduce strength training and core exercises to restore physical strength and stability.

3.3 Exercise During Midlife (36-55 Years)

Key Considerations:

- Hormonal changes due to perimenopause and menopause may lead to weight gain, reduced bone density, and muscle loss.
- Emotional health and stress management become increasingly important during this period.

Recommended Exercises:

- **Strength Training**: Weight-bearing exercises (e.g., squats, lunges, deadlifts) help prevent osteoporosis and maintain muscle mass.
- **Cardiovascular Exercise**: Moderate-intensity aerobic exercises such as brisk walking, cycling, or low-impact aerobics help maintain heart health and manage weight.
- **Flexibility and Balance Exercises**: Yoga, Pilates, and Tai Chi help maintain flexibility, balance, and mental clarity, reducing the risk of falls.
- **Pelvic Floor Exercises**: Strengthening the pelvic floor muscles through Kegel exercises can help prevent incontinence, which can be a concern as women age.

3.4 Exercise in Older Adults (55+ Years)

Key Considerations:

- Focus on maintaining independence and preventing falls.
- Exercise helps manage chronic conditions like arthritis and diabetes.

Recommended Exercises:

- **Low-Impact Cardiovascular Exercise**: Walking, swimming, and cycling are gentle on the joints while providing cardiovascular benefits.
- **Strength Training**: Light resistance training with dumbbells, resistance bands, or bodyweight exercises helps maintain muscle mass and bone density.
- **Balance and Coordination Exercises**: Tai Chi, balance training, or simple exercises like standing on one leg can help improve stability and prevent falls.
- **Flexibility Work**: Gentle stretching, yoga, or Pilates support flexibility and mobility.

1. Creating a Sustainable Fitness Routine

4.1 Setting Realistic Goals

Establishing achievable goals is essential for motivation and progress. Whether the goal is to improve cardiovascular health, build strength, or reduce stress, setting clear, measurable, and time-bound goals makes the process more manageable. Goals should be specific (e.g., walking for 30 minutes five times a week) and flexible enough to accommodate changes in circumstances.

4.2 Finding Enjoyable Activities

Sustainability in a fitness routine is primarily determined by how enjoyable the exercises are. Engaging in pleasurable activities, such as dancing, hiking, or joining a fitness class, increases adherence to the routine. Women should try different exercises to discover what they enjoy most, which will help make the routine more enjoyable and easier to stick with.

4.3 Building Consistency

Creating a regular workout schedule helps ensure consistency. The key to making exercise a habit is integrating it into daily life. To establish a routine, it may be helpful to set a fixed time each day for exercise, such as early in the morning or after work.

4.4 Progressing Gradually

Progress gradually to avoid burnout and injury. Slowly and steadily increasing the intensity, duration, or frequency of exercise over time helps the body adapt to the increased workload without causing stress or harm.

4.5 Seeking Professional Guidance

Working with a personal trainer or physical therapist can help ensure exercises are performed correctly and effectively. A fitness professional can provide tailored guidance based on individual needs, abilities, and goals.

4.6 Incorporating Rest and Recovery

Rest is an essential component of any fitness routine. Adequate rest allows muscles to repair and grow, and it helps prevent overuse injuries. Women should incorporate rest days into their fitness schedule, ensuring that their routine is balanced with time for recovery.

4.7 Staying Motivated

Tracking progress, setting new challenges, and celebrating milestones can help maintain motivation. Connecting with others through a workout buddy or group fitness class can also provide support and accountability.

Chapter 8: Hormonal Health

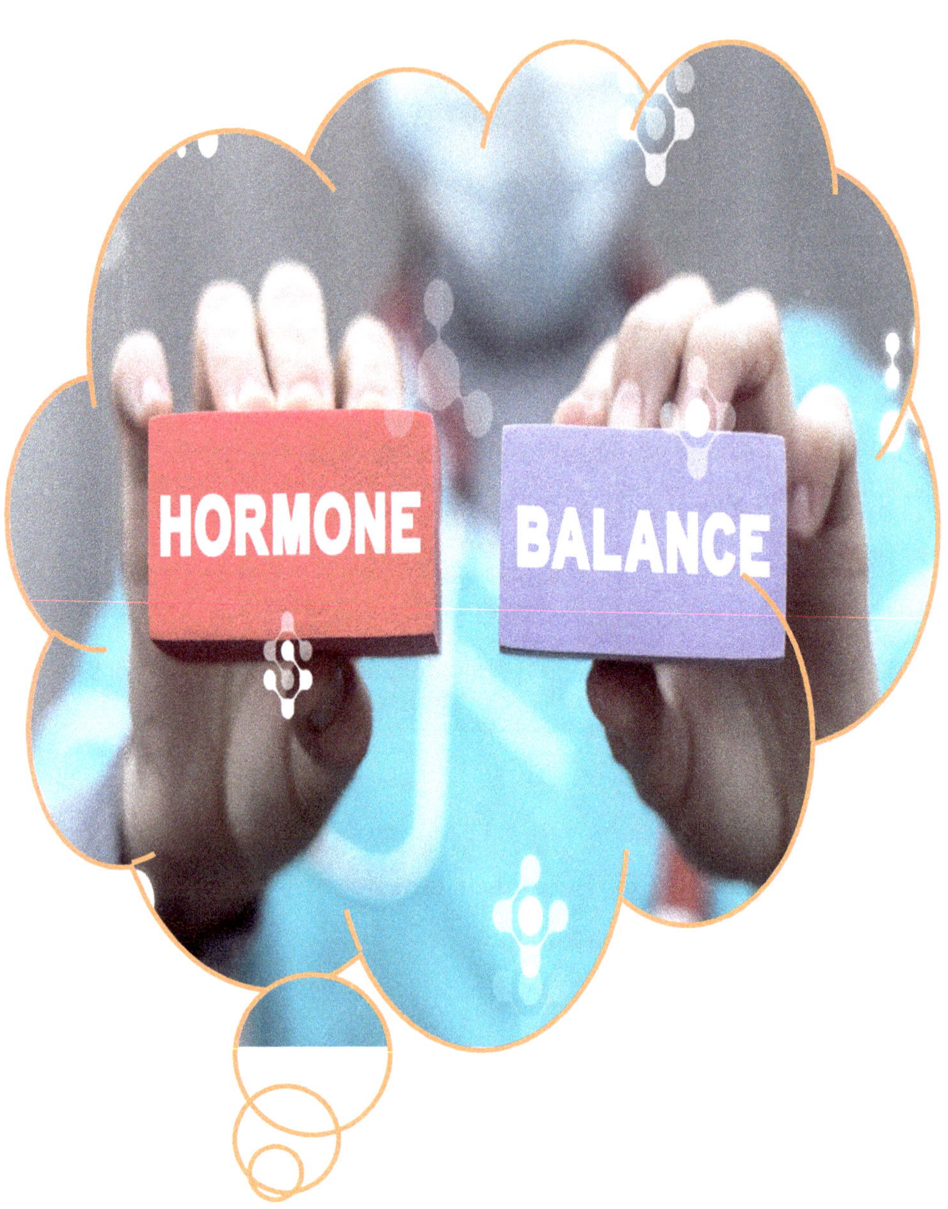

Introduction to Hormonal Health

Hormones are the body's chemical messengers. They are critical in regulating various physiological processes, including growth, metabolism, mood, and reproductive functions. Women's hormonal health is particularly crucial as they undergo significant hormonal changes throughout their lives, from puberty and pregnancy to menopause. Understanding how hormones affect women's health can empower them to take better control over their well-being.

This chapter will explore the hormones involved in women's health, common hormonal imbalances many women experience, and natural ways to support hormonal balance for overall wellness.

1. **Understanding Hormones and Their Impact on Women's Health**

Hormones are secreted by various glands in the body, including the thyroid, adrenal glands, ovaries, and pancreas. They act on specific target organs to regulate metabolism, mood, sleep, sexual function, and growth. In women, hormones significantly influence menstrual cycles, fertility, skin health, bone density, and mental well-being.

Types of Hormones:

- **Estrogen:** This primary female hormone regulates the menstrual cycle, reproductive health, and maintaining the health of bones and the cardiovascular system. Estrogen is produced mainly in the ovaries.
- **Progesterone:** This hormone works alongside estrogen and plays a key role in regulating the menstrual cycle, supporting pregnancy, and maintaining healthy estrogen levels.
- **Testosterone:** While typically considered a male hormone, women also produce small amounts of testosterone, which plays a role in libido, muscle mass, bone density, and mood.
- **Cortisol:** The adrenal glands produce the "stress hormone" cortisol. This hormone helps the body manage stress, regulate metabolism, and control blood sugar levels.
- **Thyroid Hormones (T3 and T4):** These hormones are essential for metabolism and energy production. Imbalances can result in conditions such as hypothyroidism or hyperthyroidism.
- **Insulin:** Produced by the pancreas, insulin regulates blood sugar levels and plays a role in energy storage and fat regulation.
- **Prolactin:** Produced by the pituitary gland, prolactin is essential for breast development and milk production during pregnancy and breastfeeding.

The Menstrual Cycle and Hormones

Women experience a monthly cycle of hormonal fluctuations that typically lasts around 28 days. The menstrual cycle is divided into phases: the follicular phase, ovulation, and the luteal phase. These phases are regulated by fluctuations in estrogen and progesterone levels. Hormones during these phases can affect mood, energy levels, skin, and overall well-being.

Hormones like estrogen and progesterone peak at different times during the cycle, which leads to various physical and emotional symptoms. During ovulation, estrogen peaks, leading to an increased libido and energy. In the luteal phase, progesterone rises, which can cause bloating, mood swings, and changes in appetite.

1. **Common Hormonal Imbalances and Their Symptoms**

Hormonal imbalances occur when the body produces too much or too little of a particular hormone. These imbalances can result in various symptoms that affect women's health. Some of the most common hormonal imbalances include:

a) Estrogen Dominance

Estrogen dominance occurs when the body has an excess of estrogen relative to progesterone. This imbalance can be caused by factors such as stress, poor diet, environmental toxins, and excess body fat, as fat cells can store and release estrogen.

Symptoms of Estrogen Dominance:

- Irregular or heavy periods
- PMS (premenstrual syndrome)
- Weight gain, particularly around the hips and thighs
- Mood swings and anxiety
- Fatigue and low energy
- Breast tenderness or fibrocystic breasts
- Headaches or migraines

b) Low Estrogen

Low estrogen levels can occur due to menopause, perimenopause, or other medical conditions like hypothalamic amenorrhea or ovarian failure. Estrogen plays a role in maintaining bone density, vaginal health, and cognitive function.

Symptoms of Low Estrogen:

- Hot flashes and night sweats
- Vaginal dryness and discomfort during intercourse
- Difficulty sleeping
- Memory problems and brain fog
- Decreased libido
- Dry skin and hair thinning
- Mood changes, including depression

c) Progesterone Deficiency

Progesterone deficiency occurs when the body does not produce enough progesterone, often estrogen. This imbalance can occur in the luteal phase of the menstrual cycle or during perimenopause.

Symptoms of Progesterone Deficiency:

- Irregular menstrual cycles
- Anxiety, irritability, or mood swings
- Insomnia or difficulty staying asleep
- Low libido
- Weight gain, particularly around the abdomen
- Increased risk of miscarriage (in pregnant women)

d) Polycystic Ovary Syndrome (PCOS)

PCOS is a common hormonal disorder that affects women of reproductive age. It is characterized by an imbalance in the ratio of estrogen, progesterone, and androgens (male hormones), leading to cysts on the ovaries, irregular periods, and symptoms like excess hair growth (hirsutism) and acne.

Symptoms of PCOS:

- Irregular or missed periods
- Difficulty getting pregnant
- Excess hair growth (especially on the face, chest, or back)
- Acne or oily skin
- Thinning hair on the scalp
- Weight gain or difficulty losing weight

e) Hypothyroidism (Low Thyroid Hormone)

Hypothyroidism occurs when the thyroid gland doesn't produce enough thyroid hormones (T3 and T4). The thyroid regulates metabolism, so it can slow down various bodily functions when it is underactive.

Symptoms of Hypothyroidism:

- Fatigue and lethargy
- Weight gain or difficulty losing weight
- Dry skin and hair
- Constipation
- Depression or mood swings
- Cold intolerance
- Joint pain and muscle weakness

f) Hyperthyroidism (High Thyroid Hormone)

Hyperthyroidism is the opposite of hypothyroidism, where the thyroid produces excessive amounts of hormones, speeding up metabolism.

Symptoms of Hyperthyroidism:

- Unexplained weight loss
- Rapid heartbeat or palpitations
- Anxiety or irritability
- Tremors or shaking

- Sweating and heat intolerance
- Increased appetite

g) Insulin Resistance

Insulin resistance occurs when the body's cells become less responsive to insulin, leading to elevated blood sugar levels. This condition is often linked to polycystic ovary syndrome (PCOS) and can lead to type 2 diabetes if not managed.

Symptoms of Insulin Resistance:

- Fatigue and sluggishness after meals
- Increased hunger or cravings, especially for sweets
- Weight gain, particularly around the abdomen
- Difficulty losing weight
- Increased risk of developing type 2 diabetes
- Darkened skin around the neck or armpits (acanthosis nigricans)

1. **Natural Ways to Support Hormonal Health**

Supporting hormonal health involves making lifestyle changes that promote balance and wellness. While medical intervention may be necessary in some cases, natural remedies can effectively prevent or alleviate mild hormonal imbalances.

a) Diet and Nutrition

A balanced diet rich in whole foods provides essential vitamins and minerals that support hormonal health. Key nutrients for hormone balance include:

- **Magnesium supports** adrenal health and helps balance cortisol levels. It is in dark, leafy greens, nuts, seeds, and legumes.
- **Vitamin D plays** a role in regulating estrogen levels. Sources: sunlight, fatty fish, and fortified dairy products.
- **B Vitamins,** Especially B6, B12, and folate, help regulate estrogen and progesterone levels. Sources: whole grains, legumes, lean meats, eggs.
- **Healthy Fats:** Omega-3 fatty acids support hormone production and help reduce inflammation. Sources: flaxseeds, chia seeds, walnuts, fatty fishlike salmon.
- **Fiber:** Helps regulate blood sugar levels and remove excess estrogen from the body. Sources: fruits, vegetables, whole grains, legumes.

b) Stress Management

Since cortisol, the stress hormone, significantly impacts overall hormonal balance, managing stress is crucial for hormonal health. Yoga, deep breathing, meditation, and mindfulness can help reduce stress and prevent long-term hormonal imbalances.

c) Exercise

Regular physical activity supports hormonal health by helping to regulate insulin sensitivity, balance cortisol levels, and maintain healthy body weight. Both cardiovascular exercises (walking, running, swimming) and strength training (weight lifting, resistance exercises) are beneficial.

d) Sleep Hygiene

Adequate sleep is essential for hormonal regulation. Poor sleep patterns can disrupt cortisol, melatonin, and insulin levels. Establishing a consistent sleep routine, avoiding screens before bed, and creating a calming sleep environment can improve hormonal health.

e) Herbal Remedies

Certain herbs have been traditionally used to support hormonal balance:

- **Vitex (Chaste Tree Berry):** Often used to support progesterone levels and alleviate symptoms of PMS and irregular cycles.
- **Ashwagandha:** Known for its adaptogenic properties, it helps the body manage stress and balance cortisol levels.
- **Maca Root:** Supports energy, mood, and hormone balance by acting as an adaptogen.

f) Avoiding Endocrine Disruptors

Environmental toxins, such as BPA, phthalates, and pesticides, can interfere with hormone function. Limiting exposure to these chemicals by using glass or stainless-steel containers, choosing organic foods, and avoiding plastic products can help protect hormonal health.

Conclusion

Hormonal health is a critical aspect of overall well-being.

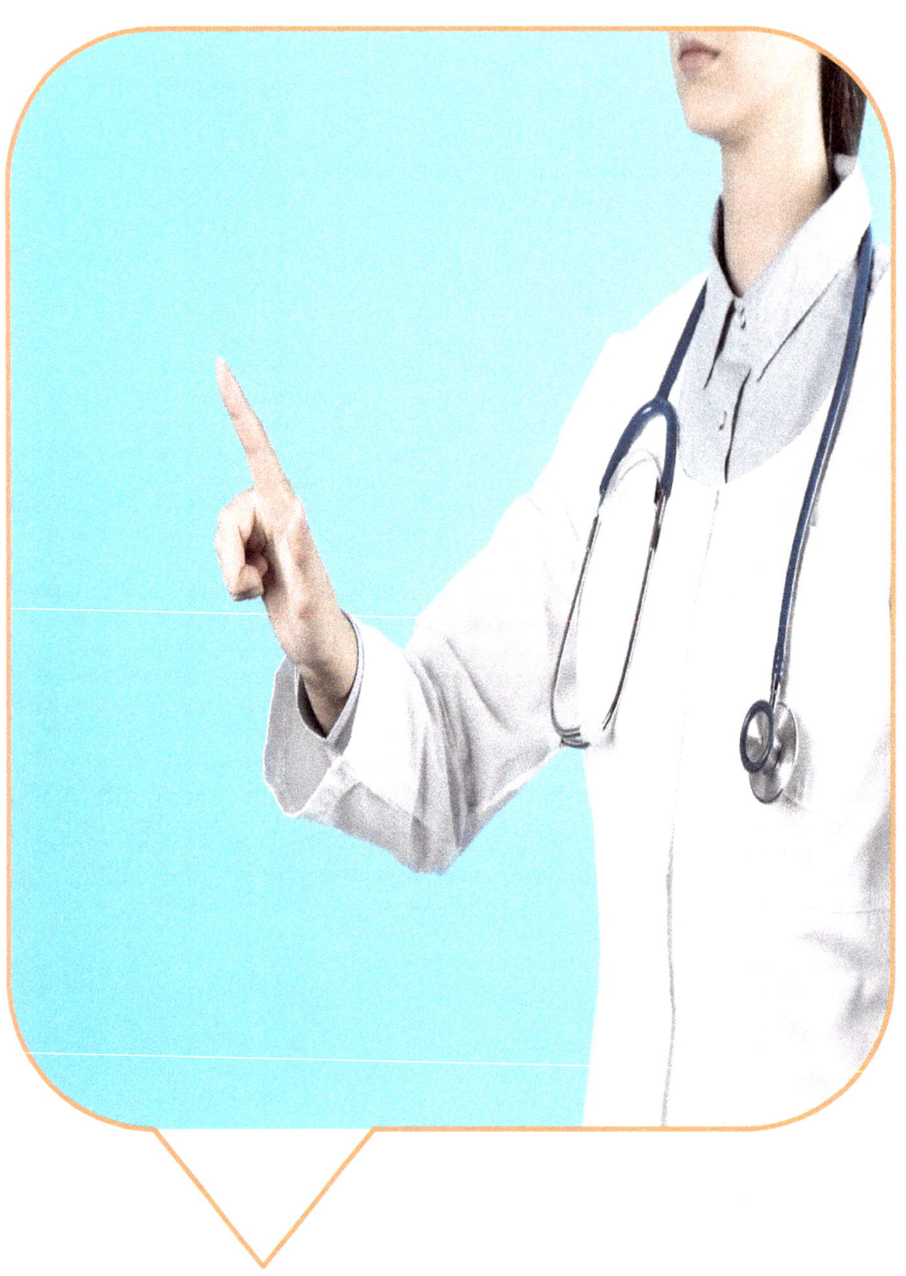

This chapter aims to empower individuals, especially women, to navigate complex healthcare systems successfully. It provides the tools, resources, and strategies for effective communication with healthcare providers, advocating for one's health needs, and accessing women-centered healthcare services. Given the significance of healthcare in everyday life, this chapter guides individuals seeking to take an active role in managing their health while understanding the nuances of healthcare delivery.

1. **Understanding How to Communicate with Healthcare Providers Effectively**
2. Importance of Communication in Healthcare

Effective communication with healthcare providers is critical to managing one's health. This sub-chapter introduces why communication is the cornerstone of quality healthcare. When patients can clearly express their symptoms, concerns, and health history, healthcare providers can offer appropriate advice, diagnosis, and treatment plans. On the flip side, when communication fails, it can lead to misdiagnosis, improper treatment, and overall dissatisfaction with care.

1. Building Trust with Your Healthcare Provider

Trust is fundamental in any healthcare relationship. A doctor-patient relationship built on mutual respect and trust enhances the likelihood of receiving personalized care. This section will explore building trust with healthcare providers, the importance of being honest about symptoms, and how patients can feel more comfortable discussing sensitive health issues.

1. Effective Communication Strategies

There are several methods and strategies for improving communication with healthcare providers:

- **Preparation before the appointment**: Writing questions and concerns beforehand helps ensure that all critical issues are discussed during the consultation.
- **Active listening**: Paying close attention to the provider's explanations and asking clarifying questions.
- **Being specific and clear**: Patients should describe their symptoms, lifestyle, and medical history as accurately as possible.
- **Use of technology**: Digital tools, such as health apps or patient portals, can help provide accurate data to healthcare providers.

Additionally, this section could delve into the role of body language, non-verbal cues, and other subtle communication methods that both the patient and provider use in these interactions.

1. Overcoming Barriers to Effective Communication

Challenges such as language differences, cultural misunderstandings, and emotional distress can affect the quality of communication in healthcare. This part addresses these barriers and offers solutions, such as:

- **Seeking interpreters or translation services** for non-native language speakers.
- **Being assertive** without being aggressive—learning to advocate for your needs while being respectful.
- **Understanding medical jargon** and asking providers to explain things in simpler terms.

1. **Tips for Advocating for Your Health**
2. The Importance of Self-Advocacy

Advocating for your health involves actively participating in your treatment process, asking questions, and seeking second opinions when necessary. This sub-chapter explains the significance of self-advocacy, especially for individuals who may feel marginalized or overlooked in healthcare settings. Women, for instance, are sometimes less likely to be taken seriously about their symptoms, so it's crucial to stand up for one's health.

1. Asserting Your Rights in Healthcare

This section will emphasize the patient's rights to:

- **Confidentiality**: Understanding the right to privacy and how healthcare providers must protect your information.
- **Informed consent**: Patients must be informed about their treatment options and have the autonomy to make decisions.
- **Access to second opinions**: Patients can seek alternative perspectives when unsure about a diagnosis.
- **Timely and respectful care**: Patients deserve care that respects their dignity and provides timely interventions.

1. Navigating Difficult Conversations with Providers

Sometimes, advocating for your health requires confronting uncomfortable topics. Whether discussing a misdiagnosis, asking for a change in treatment, or addressing concerns about a provider's behavior, this section provides practical tips for managing such situations. It could include:

- **How do you ask for clarity or further explanation?**
- **What to do if your concerns are dismissed.**
- **How to remain calm and assertive** during disagreements or frustrations with care.

1. When to Seek a Second Opinion

Seeking a second opinion can be vital, particularly when facing complex or chronic conditions. This part explains when it's appropriate to seek additional input from another healthcare provider and how to approach that conversation respectfully. It discusses the importance of gathering all relevant medical records and ensuring the second opinion is from a qualified professional.

1. Organizing Your Health Information

Staying on top of one's health data is essential to advocacy. This section will give practical advice on:

- **Creating a health portfolio**: Keeping track of medical records, prescriptions, test results, and treatment histories.
- **Using technology to manage health**: How apps and patient portals can help keep track of appointments, medications, and lab results.
- **Communicating effectively with multiple providers**: For those seeing specialists or numerous healthcare providers, coordinating care is essential to avoid miscommunication or duplication of services.

1. **Resources for Finding Women-Focused Healthcare Services**
2. Understanding Women-Centered Care

Women have unique healthcare needs, and women-centered care is designed to address those needs through comprehensive, compassionate, and respectful services. This section explores the significance of women-focused care in ensuring that women's specific health issues, such as reproductive health, mental health, and menopause, are adequately addressed.

1. National and International Resources

This sub-chapter will highlight resources available both locally and globally for women's health services:

- **National health programs**: Many countries have government-sponsored programs to provide women with affordable care.
- **International organizations**: Entities like the World Health Organization (WHO), the International Planned Parenthood Federation (IPPF), and others provide resources for women worldwide.
- **Online directories and health portals** can help women find clinics, therapists, or specialists who specialize in women's health issues.

1. Women's Health Advocacy Groups and Networks

Non-governmental organizations (NGOs) and advocacy groups can be invaluable for women seeking information about healthcare services. These groups often focus on issues such as maternal health, reproductive rights, breast cancer awareness, and women's mental health. This section will list notable organizations, their missions, and how they can assist women in finding healthcare services.

1. Finding Women-Friendly Providers

Not all healthcare providers offer women-centered care, so this section will guide you on how to:

- **Identify providers specializing in women's health**, Whether gynecologists, obstetricians, mental health professionals, or general practitioners focusing on women's health.

- **Ask the right questions**: Women should feel empowered to ask potential healthcare providers about their approach to treating women's issues.
- **Finding support for specialized needs**: This includes providers knowledgeable about LGBTQ+ health, minority women's health, and other marginalized groups.

1. Accessing Maternal and Reproductive Health Services

For women, reproductive health is a critical area where specialized services are needed. This section will address:

- **Maternity care**: Accessing prenatal and postnatal care, including the importance of prenatal vitamins, screenings, and proper birth planning.
- **Family planning**: Resources on contraception, fertility treatments, and family planning counseling.
- **Support for sexual health and well-being**: How women can find care for sexual health issues, including sexually transmitted infections, hormonal treatment, and pelvic health.

1. Telehealth and Remote Healthcare Services for Women

With the rise of telemedicine, more women are turning to remote healthcare services. This part discusses the benefits of virtual consultations, particularly for those in remote areas or who have difficulty accessing in-person care. Women can access gynecologists, mental health professionals, and general healthcare providers through online platforms.

Conclusion

Navigating healthcare systems effectively requires an understanding of one's rights, the ability to communicate effectively with healthcare providers, and the tools to advocate for one's health. This chapter provides the knowledge and resources necessary for individuals, particularly women, to confidently navigate the complexities of the healthcare system. By applying these principles, individuals can take a more active role in their health management, ensuring better outcomes and greater satisfaction with their healthcare experiences.

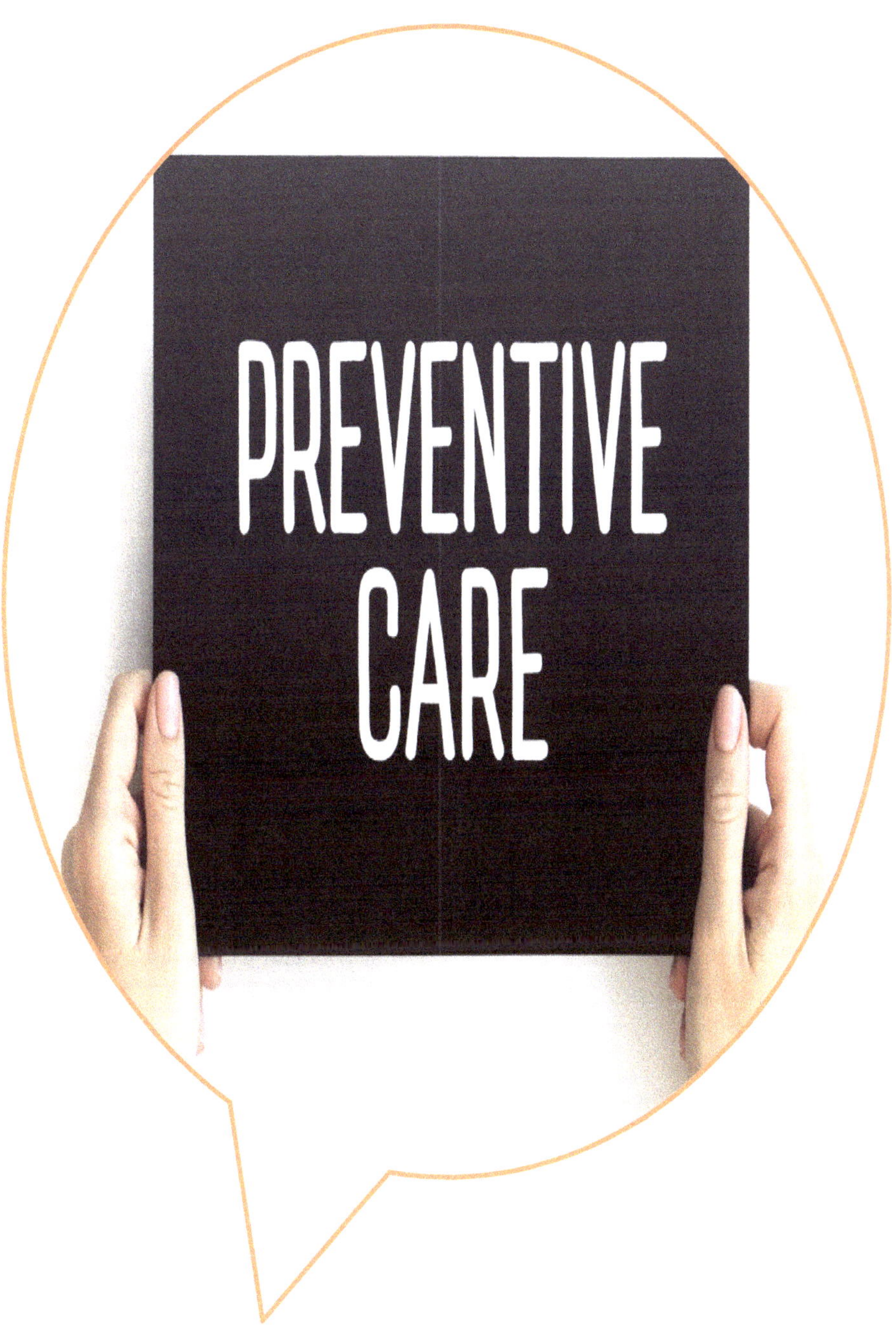
PREVENTIVE
CARE

Introduction

Preventive care and screenings are vital aspects of maintaining good health and preventing diseases before they occur or in their early stages. An intense preventive care regimen can help ensure longer, healthier lives for women who face unique health challenges at different life stages. This chapter explores the importance of preventive care in women's health, outlines key recommended screenings and vaccinations, and offers guidance on creating a personalized preventive care plan.

1. Importance of Preventive Care in Women's Health

Preventive care refers to the actions taken to prevent illness or disease rather than waiting for symptoms to appear. This means focusing on early detection, health promotion, and risk reduction strategies for women. Here are key reasons why preventive care is essential:

1.1. Early Detection of Diseases

Many chronic diseases, such as cancer, heart disease, and diabetes, can be asymptomatic in the early stages. Regular screenings can detect these conditions early when they are easier to treat and manage. For example, mammograms for breast cancer or Pap smears for cervical cancer can lead to earlier diagnoses, which can significantly improve outcomes.

1.2. Health Promotion

Preventive care emphasizes healthy lifestyles, such as maintaining a balanced diet, regular physical activity, stress management, and proper sleep. By adopting these habits early in life, women can reduce the risk of chronic conditions like obesity, hypertension, and osteoporosis.

1.3. Reducing Healthcare Costs

Preventing the onset of diseases and detecting them early can reduce healthcare costs over time. Treating conditions in their early stages is generally less expensive than treating them when they are more advanced, requiring more intensive care and possibly hospitalization.

1.4. Personalized Approach

Preventive care considers the unique health needs of women at different ages, from adolescence through menopause and beyond. Women's health varies depending on hormonal changes, reproductive health, and genetics. A personalized preventive care plan considers these factors and ensures that health screenings are tailored to an individual's needs.

1.5. Empowerment

Women can feel more empowered and involved in their health decisions by taking charge of their health. Preventive care encourages women to be proactive, which leads to better outcomes and higher satisfaction with healthcare services.

1. Recommended Screenings and Vaccinations

Screenings and vaccinations are cornerstone practices in preventive care. Specific screenings are recommended for women based on age, risk factors, and family history. Here is an overview of the most common screenings and vaccinations for women:

2.1. Cancer Screenings

Cancer is one of the leading causes of death for women, but early detection through screenings can save lives. The following are critical screenings for various types of cancer:

- **Breast Cancer Screening:**
    - Mammography: Women aged 50 to 74 should have mammograms every two years, though earlier screenings may be recommended for those with a family history of breast cancer.
    - Clinical Breast Exam: Women should perform regular self-exams and have a clinical breast exam (CBE) during routine check-ups to detect lumps or changes.
- **Cervical Cancer Screening:**
    - Pap Smear: Starting at age 21, women should undergo Pap smears every three years to detect abnormal cells that could develop into cervical cancer.
    - HPV Testing: Women over 30 should undergo co-testing with Pap smears and HPV testing every five years.
- **Colorectal Cancer Screening:**
    - Colonoscopy: Recommended for women starting at age 50, with follow-up screenings every 10 years or earlier if there's a family history of colorectal cancer or other risk factors.

2.2. Cardiovascular Disease Screenings

Heart disease is the leading cause of death among women. Regular screenings for heart disease risk factors are crucial.

- **Blood Pressure Screening**: High blood pressure is a significant risk factor for heart disease. Starting at age 20, women should have their blood pressure checked at least once every two years.
- **Cholesterol Screening**: Women aged 45 and older should have their cholesterol levels checked every 4–6 years. Those at higher risk may need more frequent testing.
- **Blood Glucose Screening**: Women with risk factors for diabetes, such as obesity or a family history of diabetes, should undergo blood glucose screening regularly.

2.3. Bone Health Screenings

As women age, they become more prone to osteoporosis, a condition where bones become fragile and more prone to fractures.

- **Bone Density Test (DEXA Scan)**: Women over 65 or younger with risk factors such as a family history or prior fractures should measure their bone density to assess their osteoporosis risk.

2.4. Sexual and Reproductive Health Screenings

- **STI Testing**: Women should undergo testing for sexually transmitted infections (STIs) based on their sexual activity and risk factors. This is particularly important for those under 25 or those with multiple partners.
- **Pelvic Exams**: Women should have a pelvic exam as part of their annual gynecological check-up to detect any reproductive health issues, such as ovarian cysts or fibroids.

2.5. Mental Health Screenings

Mental health is a critical component of overall well-being, and regular screenings can help identify conditions such as depression and anxiety.

- **Depression Screening**: Women should be screened for depression during routine medical exams, especially if they have risk factors like a history of mental health disorders, pregnancy complications, or significant life stressors.

2.6. Vaccinations

Vaccines are essential to prevent a range of illnesses. Key vaccinations for women include:

- **Human Papillomavirus (HPV) Vaccine**: Recommended for girls and young women aged 11–26 to prevent cervical cancer and other HPV-related cancers.
- **Flu Vaccine**: Annual flu shots are recommended for all women, especially during pregnancy and those with chronic health conditions.
- **Tetanus, Diphtheria, and Pertussis (Tdap) Vaccine**: This vaccine is recommended for pregnant women during each pregnancy to protect both mother and newborn from whooping cough.
- **Hepatitis B Vaccine**: Women at risk of hepatitis B, particularly those with multiple sexual partners or healthcare workers, should receive the vaccine.

1. **How to Create a Personalized Preventive Care Plan**

A personalized preventive care plan is tailored to an individual's unique health needs, risk factors, and goals. Here's how to create one:

3.1. Assess Personal Health History

The first step in developing a personalized care plan is to assess a woman's health history, including any family history of diseases such as cancer, heart disease, diabetes, or mental health conditions. This helps identify risk areas that may require more frequent or specialized screenings.

3.2. Consider Age and Life Stage

Preventive care needs to change over a woman's lifetime. A young woman's plan may focus on reproductive health and STI screening, while a woman in her 40s may need to focus on heart health and breast cancer screenings. A post-menopausal woman may need to concentrate on bone health and colorectal cancer screenings.

3.3. Lifestyle and Risk Factors

Lifestyle choices play a huge role in preventive health. A woman's diet, physical activity, alcohol consumption, and smoking habits must be considered. Women with high-risk factors, such as obesity, a sedentary lifestyle, or a history of substance abuse, may need more intensive screenings or interventions.

3.4. Collaborate with Healthcare Providers

Developing a personalized preventive care plan should involve collaboration with healthcare providers, such as a primary care physician, gynecologist, or cardiologist. These professionals can provide guidance on necessary screenings, vaccines, and lifestyle changes.

3.5. Set Specific Health Goals

Specific goals should be set once a woman's health risks and needs are identified. These may include maintaining a healthy weight, managing cholesterol levels, scheduling annual check-ups, or ensuring that necessary screenings are up to date.

3.6. Follow-up and Monitoring

A key component of any preventive care plan is monitoring progress. Regular follow-up appointments are essential to assess whether goals are being met and to make any necessary adjustments. This ensures that women remain proactive in managing their health.

3.7. Empowerment through Education

Educating women about their health and the importance of preventive care is crucial. This includes helping them understand the screenings and vaccines recommended for their age group and encouraging them to be proactive in making health decisions.

Conclusion

Preventive care is a cornerstone of women's health, offering numerous benefits, including early disease detection, improved health outcomes, and lower healthcare costs. By understanding the importance of regular screenings and vaccinations and creating personalized care plans, women can take proactive steps to safeguard their health at every stage of life. Empowering women through education and collaboration with healthcare providers enables them to make informed decisions that will help lead to a longer, healthier life.

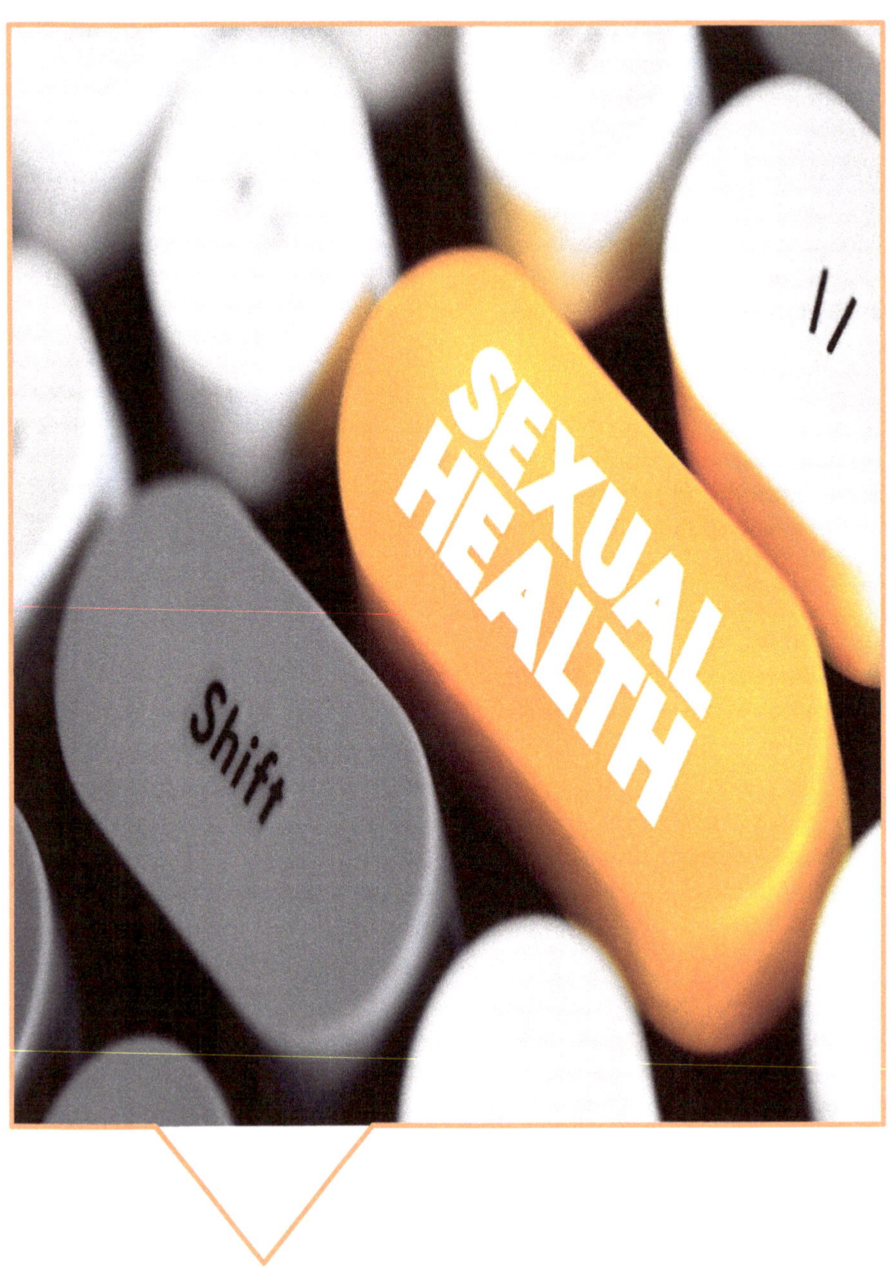

SEXUAL HEALTH
Shift

Introduction to Sexual Health and Wellness

Sexual health is a critical aspect of an individual's overall well-being. It encompasses physical, emotional, mental, and social health about sexuality. A comprehensive understanding of sexual health is essential not only for preventing sexual health problems but also for fostering fulfilling and safe sexual experiences. Sexual wellness is linked with positive sexual experiences and a healthy attitude toward one's body, relationships, and sexual behaviors. It goes beyond the absence of disease or dysfunction and includes the ability to enjoy and express one's sexuality safely and responsibly.

In this chapter, we explore the multifaceted aspects of sexual health and wellness, discuss common sexual health issues, and delve into the best practices for maintaining sexual health, including communication, consent, and safe sexual practices. The chapter also highlights how personal values, cultural context, and societal influences impact sexual health, making it a diverse and evolving field.

1. **Understanding Sexual Health and Its Importance**

Sexual health is often overlooked or underappreciated in medical and psychological discussions, but it plays a fundamental role in our overall health and happiness. The **World Health Organization (WHO)** defines sexual health as a state of physical, emotional, mental, and social well-being about sexuality. This definition stresses that sexual health is more than just the absence of sexual dysfunctions or diseases; it includes positive and respectful sexual relationships, access to sexual education, and the ability to express one's sexuality without harm, coercion, or discrimination.

1.1 Physical Aspects of Sexual Health

The physical dimension of sexual health refers to the physiological functions of the sexual organs and reproductive system. This includes regular menstruation, the ability to engage in sexual activity comfortably, and maintaining reproductive health. It involves understanding and addressing common sexual dysfunctions such as erectile dysfunction (ED), vaginal dryness, and painful intercourse. Regular medical check-ups and preventive measures, such as screening for sexually transmitted infections (STIs), also form an integral part of physical sexual health.

1.2 Emotional and Mental Well-being

Emotional well-being is just as crucial as physical health in sexual health. A person's emotional state can significantly impact their sexual desires, satisfaction, and performance. Feelings of shame, guilt, or anxiety about one's body or sexual orientation can hinder one's ability to engage in healthy sexual relationships. Mental health disorders such as depression or anxiety may also affect sexual health, leading to decreased libido, avoidance of sexual intimacy, or sexual dysfunction.

Mental wellness also involves an individual's understanding of their sexual preferences, desires, and boundaries, leading to better communication and more positive sexual experiences.

1.3 Social and Cultural Context

Sexual health does not exist in a vacuum; the social, cultural, and political environment influences it. Societal norms around gender, sexuality, and relationships play a role in shaping how individuals view their sexual health. For example, cultures that prioritize specific values, such as abstinence before marriage, may lead to a person feeling conflicted about their sexual desires, leading to shame or repression. Conversely, cultures that promote sexual freedom may encourage healthier attitudes but may also risk be neglecting sexual responsibility and consent.

Moreover, access to sexual education, health services, and supportive communities can determine how individuals manage their sexual health. In some parts of the world, sexual health resources may be limited, leading to higher rates of unplanned pregnancies, STIs, and sexual violence.

1. **Common Sexual Health Issues and Concerns**

Many individuals face sexual health challenges throughout their lives. These issues can vary based on age, gender, sexual orientation, and life experiences. Addressing these concerns is crucial to ensuring individuals maintain a healthy and positive relationship with their sexuality.

2.1 Sexually Transmitted Infections (STIs)

STIs are infections that are commonly transmitted through sexual contact. They can affect both men and women and may have long-term health consequences if left untreated. The most common STIs include **chlamydia, gonorrhea, syphilis, herpes**, and **HIV/AIDS**.

Prevention through safe sexual practices, such as the use of condoms and regular testing, is essential for managing sexual health. Many STIs can be asymptomatic, meaning they may not show symptoms even if a person is infected. This is why routine screenings and communication with sexual partners are critical.

2.2 Sexual Dysfunction

Sexual dysfunction refers to the inability to enjoy sexual activity or experience sexual satisfaction. Both men and women can experience sexual dysfunction, which can include issues like:

- **Erectile dysfunction** (ED): Inability to achieve or maintain an erection sufficient for sexual activity.
- **Low libido**: Reduced desire for sexual activity, often linked to hormonal imbalances, emotional stress, or relationship issues.
- **Anorgasmia**: Difficulty achieving orgasm despite adequate sexual stimulation.

These dysfunctions can have various causes, including physical, psychological, and relational factors. Treatment options depend on the underlying cause and may include therapy, medication, or lifestyle changes.

2.3 Contraception and Family Planning

One of the most common sexual health concerns for individuals and couples is the management of contraception and family planning. Unplanned pregnancies, for example, can have significant personal, social, and economic consequences. Access to a range of contraceptive methods — including birth control pills, condoms, intrauterine devices (IUDs), and sterilization — is essential for sexual health and empowerment.

Choosing the proper contraception method depends on individual health needs, lifestyle, and personal preferences. Medical professionals can guide individuals in selecting the most appropriate contraception methods, taking into account factors like health risks, ease of use, and reliability.

2.4 Sexual Abuse and Violence

Sexual violence and abuse are grave concerns for sexual health, as they often lead to long-term psychological and physical harm. Survivors of sexual abuse may experience trauma, anxiety, depression, and PTSD, which can affect their sexual relationships and general well-being. Addressing sexual abuse requires comprehensive support systems, including counseling, legal aid, and medical assistance.

In many societies, issues such as **rape culture**, harassment, and coercion persist, and these can perpetuate harmful norms about consent and boundaries. Education around consent, communication, and respect is crucial in reducing sexual violence and improving sexual health outcomes.

2.5 Body Image and Self-Esteem

Body image issues often affect sexual health, particularly in individuals who feel dissatisfaction with their physical appearance. This can lead to reduced confidence, reluctance to engage in sexual activity, or anxiety during intimate moments. Developing a positive body image and self-esteem is critical for overall sexual wellness. Therapy, mindfulness, and body-positive movements are key resources in promoting healthier attitudes toward one's body and sexuality.

1. **Safe Practices and Communication in Sexual Relationships**

Maintaining sexual health involves more than just addressing medical issues; it is also about practicing safe sexual behaviors and fostering open communication in relationships. Ensuring that sexual activity is consensual, secure, and respectful is fundamental to both individual well-being and collective sexual wellness.

3.1 Consent and Communication

One of the foundational principles of healthy sexual relationships is **consent**. Consent refers to a voluntary, clear, and enthusiastic agreement between all parties involved in sexual activity. Effective communication is vital for ensuring that consent is given and respected.

Open dialogue about desires, boundaries, and preferences helps create a safe and respectful environment where both partners feel heard and valued. This includes discussions about contraception, safe sex practices, and any concerns or fears regarding sexual health.

3.2 Condom Use and Safe Sex Practices

The most effective way to prevent sexually transmitted infections (STIs) and unplanned pregnancies during sexual activity is to use **condoms** correctly and consistently. In addition to condoms, **dental dams** can be used for oral sex, and other barrier methods can be used depending on the type of sexual activity.

It is also essential to recognize that not all sexual acts carry the same level of risk for STIs, but practicing safer sex, such as limiting the number of sexual partners and getting regular health check-ups, is key.

3.3 Regular Health Check-Ups

A proactive approach to sexual health involves regular check-ups with healthcare providers. These can include STI screenings, pelvic exams, mammograms (for women), and prostate exams (for men), as well as discussions about contraception and reproductive health.

Routine testing helps identify potential health issues before they become serious, and it promotes sexual wellness by ensuring individuals are informed and able to make decisions about their sexual health.

3.4 Healthy Relationship Practices

Sexual health does not exist in isolation but is deeply intertwined with the quality of intimate relationships. Healthy relationships are characterized by trust, mutual respect, and shared responsibility for sexual health. Couples should regularly communicate about their sexual needs, desires, and boundaries. Moreover, they should support one another in making informed decisions about contraception, STI testing, and safe sex practices.

In situations where there are issues such as infidelity, coercion, or abuse, seeking professional help can provide the tools necessary to rebuild or move on from unhealthy dynamics.

Conclusion

Sexual health is integral to overall well-being, influencing physical, emotional, mental, and social health. Understanding sexual health involves acknowledging the complexity of sexual experiences and addressing the challenges that may arise from cultural, medical, or relational factors. By fostering open communication, practicing safe behaviors, and maintaining an informed approach to sexual health, individuals can lead healthier and more fulfilling sexual lives.

Education, accessibility to healthcare, and mutual respect are essential elements in improving sexual health outcomes for all individuals. As society continues to evolve, it is crucial to continue promoting comprehensive, inclusive, and evidence-based sexual health education to ensure a healthier future for all.

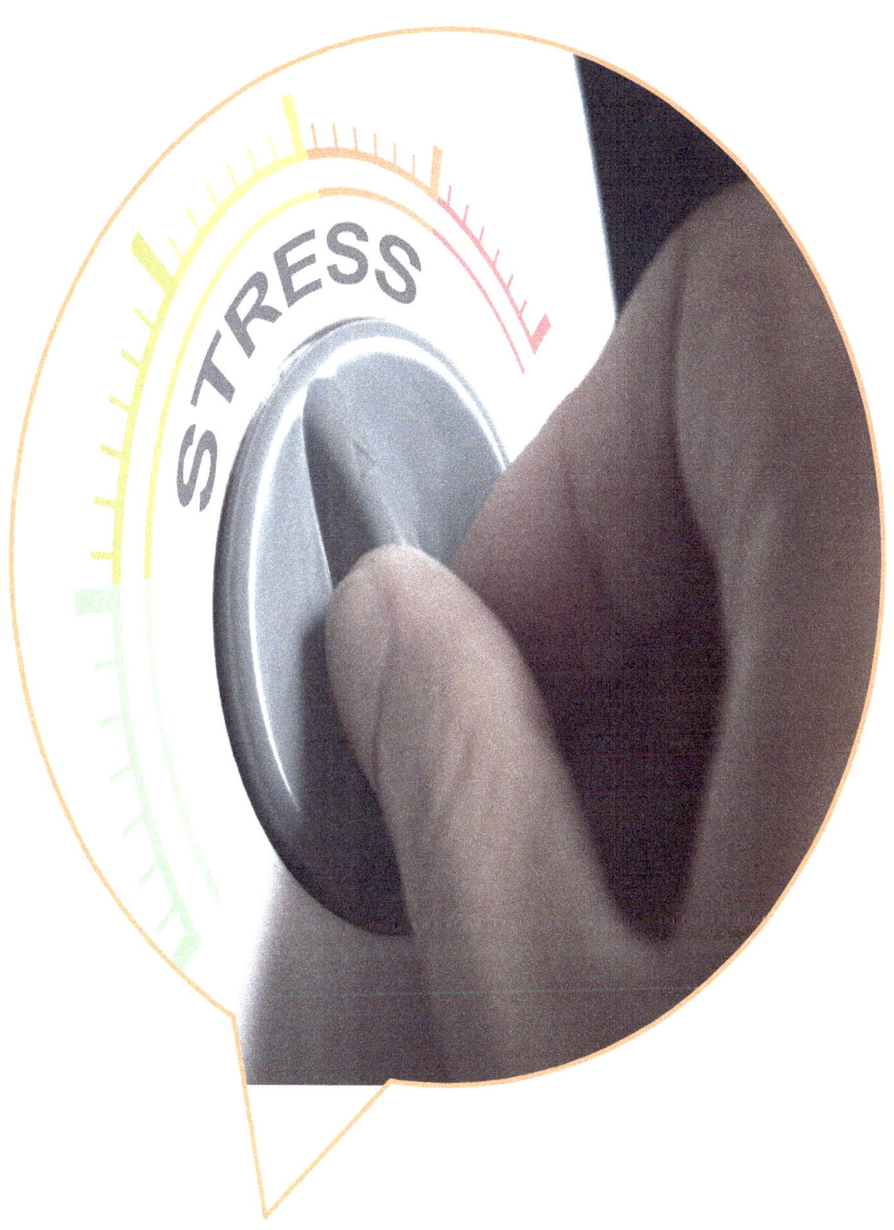
STRESS

Stress and burnout are increasingly common challenges women face, often due to the balancing act of multiple roles in both personal and professional spheres. This chapter explores the sources of stress in women's lives, offers techniques for stress management and relaxation, and highlights the importance of self-care and boundary-setting to mitigate the impact of stress.

1. Identifying Sources of Stress in Women's Lives

1.1 Workplace Stress

The modern workplace presents a range of stressors, from heavy workloads to unclear job expectations. Women often face unique challenges in the workplace, such as gender biases, unequal pay, or expectations to prove themselves in male-dominated fields. Workplace stress can result from long hours, job insecurity, and lack of support or recognition.

In addition, the increasing prevalence of remote work, while offering flexibility, can also blur the boundaries between personal and professional lives. Women may feel pressure to be constantly available, leading to burnout.

1.2 Family and Caregiving Responsibilities

Women are often primary caregivers in families, balancing the responsibilities of parenting, household chores, and caring for elderly relatives. This caregiving burden can cause physical, emotional, and mental exhaustion. The constant juggling between work and family commitments can lead to feelings of guilt and inadequacy, further exacerbating stress levels.

In many cultures, societal expectations squarely place the responsibility of caregiving on women's shoulders, even in households where both partners work. The disproportionate distribution of unpaid labor at home can lead to frustration, resentment, and stress.

1.3 Social and Cultural Pressures

Social expectations, such as the pressure to conform to specific beauty standards or roles, can create significant stress. Women often experience pressure to "have it all" – a fulfilling career, a successful family life, and a specific physical appearance. This idealized image of womanhood can cause anxiety and self-esteem issues when women are unable to meet these societal standards.

Moreover, women may face stress from cultural expectations regarding their behavior, career choices, or independence. In many societies, women are expected to sacrifice personal desires for the good of their families, contributing to stress and feelings of being overwhelmed.

1.4 Financial Stress

Financial insecurity is a significant source of stress for women, particularly for single mothers or women in lower-income households. The gender pay gap further compounds this issue, as women may struggle to achieve financial independence. Financial worries can have a far-reaching impact, affecting overall well-being, health, and family dynamics.

Women in precarious financial situations may experience chronic anxiety, which can eventually manifest in physical symptoms like insomnia, headaches, or digestive problems. The fear of being unable to meet financial obligations or provide for dependents creates immense stress.

1.5 Health Concerns

Health-related stress is a significant concern for many women. Issues such as reproductive health, menopause, and the constant juggling of health needs, often combined with a demanding lifestyle, can lead to stress. The fear of chronic illness, aging, or the physical toll of caregiving can further heighten anxiety.

Women also face a higher risk of developing mental health conditions, such as depression and anxiety, due to hormonal fluctuations, societal pressures, and the demands of caregiving roles.

1. Techniques for Stress Management and Relaxation

2.1 Mindfulness and Meditation

Mindfulness is being fully present at the moment, acknowledging and accepting feelings without judgment. Mindfulness exercises, such as meditation, deep breathing, and body scanning, help reduce stress by promoting a state of calm and relaxation. These techniques can help women manage overwhelming emotions, such as anxiety, fear, and guilt.

Regular mindfulness encourages individuals to focus on their immediate experience rather than worrying about past or future events. This reduces mental clutter and fosters a sense of peace and well-being. Incorporating mindfulness into daily routines, such as morning meditation or guided imagery, can significantly alleviate stress.

2.2 Physical Exercise and Movement

Exercise is one of the most effective ways to combat stress. Physical activity releases endorphins, the body's natural mood boosters. Women who engage in regular exercise, whether jogging, yoga, swimming or even dancing, can experience significant reductions in stress levels.

Yoga, in particular, has gained recognition for its ability to promote relaxation and reduce tension. It combines physical movement with breathing exercises, which help to relax the body and clear the mind. Women can also use exercise as a form of self-care, using time for physical activity to reconnect with their bodies and release built-up stress.

2.3 Breathing Exercises

Breathing techniques, such as diaphragmatic breathing, box breathing, or alternate nostril breathing, can help women manage acute stress. The body shifts from the "fight-or-flight" stress response to a more relaxed, parasympathetic state by consciously slowing down the breath and focusing on deep inhalations and exhalations.

Practicing deep breathing for just a few minutes can lower blood pressure, reduce anxiety, and create a sense of calm. This technique can be used anytime, anywhere – at work, home, or even during social interactions – to manage stress levels.

2.4 Progressive Muscle Relaxation (PMR)

PMR involves tensing and then relaxing different muscle groups in the body. This practice helps women become more aware of areas in their bodies where they hold tension and allows them to relax those muscles consciously. PMR is beneficial for stress relief, as it helps release physical tension that builds up during periods of high stress.

Women can feel more grounded and relaxed by progressively moving through each muscle group. Regular practice of PMR can reduce chronic pain, improve sleep, and provide long-term benefits for managing stress.

2.5 Creative Outlets

Engaging in creative activities, such as painting, drawing, writing, or crafting, can be a therapeutic way to manage stress. Creativity provides a mental escape, allowing women to express emotions and thoughts that may be difficult to articulate. Art and creative writing, in particular, help release pent-up feelings and provide a healthy way to cope with stress.

Journaling, for instance, allows individuals to process and reflect on their emotions, which can help release anxiety and improve mental clarity. Creating something tangible can provide a sense of accomplishment, improve self-esteem, and reduce stress.

2.6 Social Support and Connection

Building a strong support network is essential for stress management. Women who feel connected to others, whether through close friends, family, or support groups, tend to experience less stress than those who feel isolated. Talking about worries with a trusted individual can provide emotional relief and help reframe challenges in a more manageable way.

In addition to peer support, professional counseling or therapy may also be valuable for addressing deeper stressors or chronic burnout. Cognitive-behavioral therapy (CBT) is a widely used approach to helping women develop healthier thought patterns and coping mechanisms to manage stress.

2.7 Time Management and Organization

Poor time management can be a major contributor to stress. Women juggling multiple roles may be overwhelmed by deadlines, household tasks, or social obligations. Learning effective time management techniques, such as creating to-do lists, setting realistic goals, and breaking tasks into smaller, more manageable steps, can significantly reduce stress.

Time management tools, such as digital calendars or productivity apps, help women stay on track and prioritize tasks, reducing feelings of chaos or helplessness. Organizing time effectively gives women more control over their schedules and helps prevent stress from spiraling out of control.

1. ## The Importance of Self-Care and Setting Boundaries

3.1 Defining Self-Care

Self-care refers to activities and practices that women engage in to maintain their mental, emotional, and physical health. These practices are vital in reducing stress and preventing burnout. Unfortunately, many women neglect self-care due to busy schedules, feelings of guilt, or societal pressures. However, prioritizing self-care is essential for maintaining long-term well-being.

Self-care can be as simple as taking a relaxing bath, reading a book, or spending time in nature. It involves setting aside time to replenish one's energy and focus on personal well-being. Practicing self-care regularly helps reduce the harmful effects of stress and improves overall quality of life.

3.2 Setting Boundaries

Setting clear boundaries is crucial for managing stress. Women often struggle with saying "no" due to cultural expectations or the fear of letting others down. However, overcommitting to responsibilities can lead to burnout and exhaustion. Learning to set and communicate boundaries with family, friends, and coworkers is essential for preserving personal energy.

Healthy boundaries involve recognizing one's limits and making space for self-care, relaxation, and personal interests. This might include limiting work hours, not taking on additional caregiving roles, or setting boundaries in social relationships. By maintaining these boundaries, women can prevent stress from taking over their lives and create a healthier balance between personal and professional demands.

3.3 Prioritizing Personal Well-being

Women often prioritize the needs of others before their own, which can lead to neglect of their well-being. Prioritizing personal well-being involves acknowledging the need for rest, relaxation, and time alone. It also means recognizing when stress is unmanageable and taking proactive steps to address it.

Prioritizing their health can better equip women to care for others and perform well in their various roles. Regular breaks, healthy eating, and sufficient sleep contribute to a more balanced and less stressful life.

3.4 Building Resilience

Resilience is the ability to adapt and bounce back from adversity. Building resilience is an ongoing process that helps women cope with stress and prevent burnout. Developing resilience involves fostering a positive mindset and seeking support when needed.

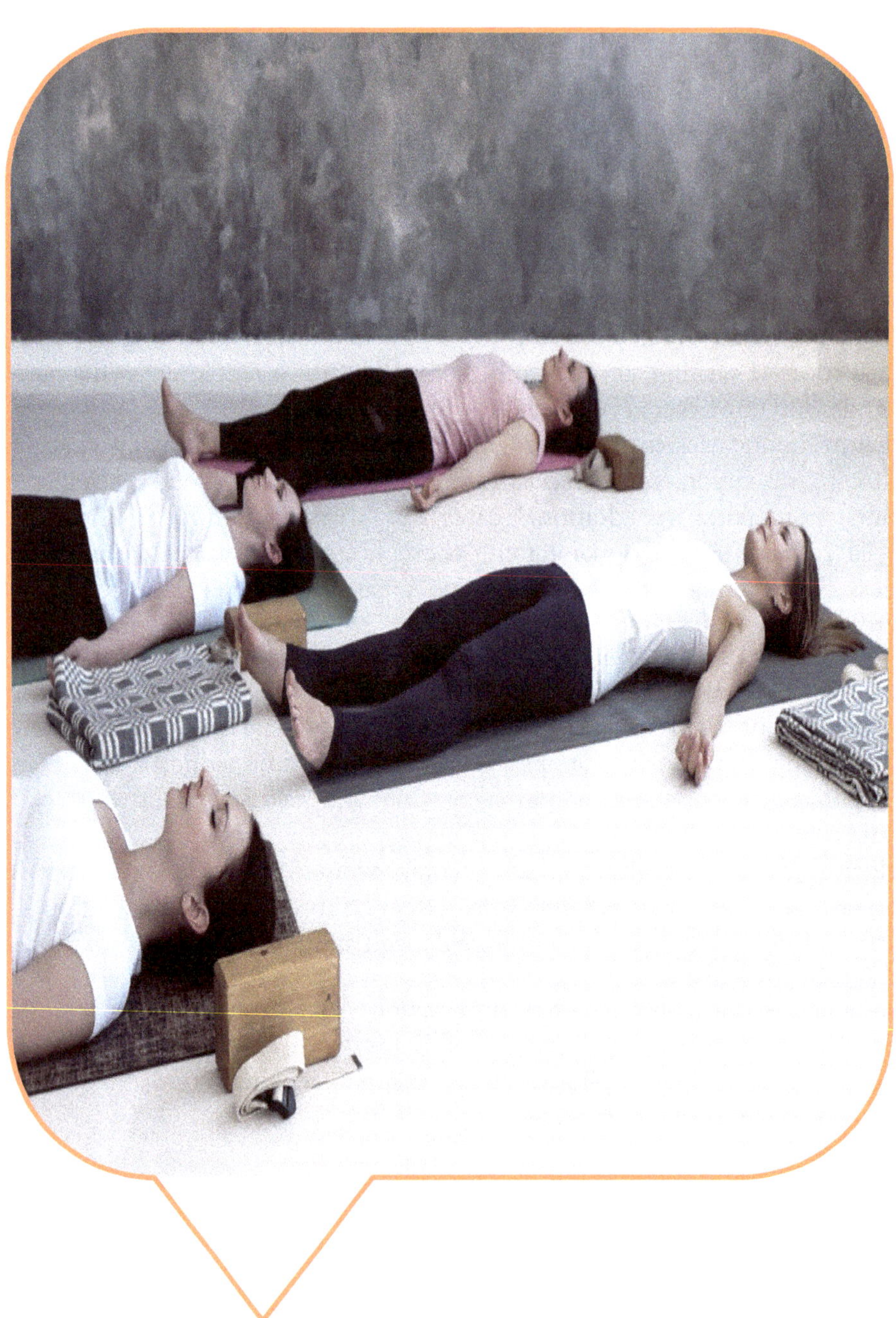

The Role of Sleep in Overall Health

Sleep is an essential, biologically driven behavior necessary for physical and mental health. Although it is often overlooked or undervalued in today's fast-paced society, sleep is a cornerstone of overall well-being. Sleep serves multiple critical functions, from restoring energy levels to enhancing cognitive function and immune response. In this section, we will delve into sleep's multifaceted role in maintaining good health.

1. **Physical Restoration and Energy Regulation**

One of the primary roles of sleep is physical restoration. During sleep, the body undergoes processes that repair cells, restore muscle tissue, and rejuvenate the organs. This is particularly important for women, who may have differing sleep needs due to hormonal fluctuations at different points in their lives. Sleep helps regulate the body's energy balance and contributes to maintaining a healthy weight. Lack of sleep has been associated with increased hunger and cravings for high-calorie foods, which can contribute to weight gain.

1. **Cognitive Function and Memory Consolidation**

Sleep is crucial for cognitive functioning. During sleep, especially during rapid eye movement (REM), the brain processes and consolidates memories from the day. Sleep allows the brain to connect new information and pre-existing knowledge, enhancing learning and creativity. It also helps in clearing metabolic waste products, including amyloid-beta, which is associated with Alzheimer's disease. The result is better decision-making, problem-solving, and the ability to manage stress, which is fundamental to a person's overall quality of life.

1. **Mental Health and Emotional Regulation**

Sleep plays a significant role in emotional regulation. Chronic sleep deprivation is linked to a range of mental health issues, including anxiety, depression, and irritability. For women who may face higher rates of mood disorders due to hormonal fluctuations, ensuring adequate sleep is a preventive measure against emotional distress. During sleep, the brain processes emotional experiences, helping to manage stress and reduce emotional reactivity. Sufficient sleep improves resilience to mental health challenges and enhances mood stability.

1. **Immune System Function**

Sleep is critical to the immune system's function. During sleep, the body produces immune cells and proteins, including cytokines. These substances help the body fight infections and inflammation. Sleep deprivation has been shown to weaken the immune system, making individuals more susceptible to illnesses such as colds and infections. This is particularly significant for women during pregnancy, menopause, or times of increased stress when immune function might be compromised.

1. **Hormonal Regulation and Reproductive Health**

For women, sleep plays a crucial role in hormonal balance. Hormones such as cortisol, estrogen, and progesterone are regulated during sleep cycles. For example, cortisol (the stress hormone) decreases during sleep, allowing the body to recover from the day's stresses. Disruptions in sleep, especially chronic sleep deprivation, can lead to hormonal imbalances that affect reproductive health, menstrual cycles, and fertility. Furthermore, sleep patterns can influence the severity of symptoms during perimenopause and menopause, such as hot flashes, sleep disturbances, and mood swings.

Common Sleep Disorders Affecting Women

While sleep is essential for health, many women experience sleep disorders that can disrupt their overall well-being. These disorders may be caused by various factors, including hormonal changes, lifestyle stressors, and underlying health conditions. Here, we examine some of the most common sleep disorders that affect women.

1. **Insomnia**

Insomnia is one of the most common sleep disorders, characterized by difficulty falling asleep or staying asleep or waking up too early without being able to return to sleep. Women are more likely than men to experience insomnia, particularly during pregnancy, perimenopause, and menopause, due to fluctuating hormone levels. Stress, anxiety, depression, and poor sleep habits also contribute to insomnia. The impact of insomnia can be profound, affecting cognitive performance, emotional regulation, and overall health.

1. **Sleep Apnea**

Sleep apnea is a disorder that causes interrupted breathing during sleep. The most common type of sleep apnea is obstructive sleep apnea (OSA), where the airway becomes blocked, leading to pauses in breathing throughout the night. Women are less likely than men to develop sleep apnea, but it is still a significant concern, especially during menopause. Hormonal changes, weight gain, and other risk factors can contribute to the onset of sleep apnea in women. Symptoms include snoring, gasping for air during sleep, excessive daytime sleepiness, and difficulty concentrating. Sleep apnea can lead to increased risks of cardiovascular disease, hypertension, and diabetes.

1. **Restless Leg Syndrome (RLS)**

Restless Leg Syndrome (RLS) is a neurological condition that causes an uncontrollable urge to move the legs, typically accompanied by uncomfortable sensations. These symptoms worsen during inactivity, especially in the evening or at night, making it difficult to fall asleep. RLS is more common in women, particularly during pregnancy, and can be exacerbated by hormonal changes, iron deficiency, or certain medications. The discomfort and need to move the legs can significantly impair the ability to sleep properly.

1. **Narcolepsy**

Narcolepsy is a chronic sleep disorder characterized by excessive daytime sleepiness and sudden, uncontrollable sleep attacks. Women may experience narcolepsy differently from men, with more frequent symptoms in adolescence or early adulthood. The condition can severely impact daily life and social interactions. In addition to daytime sleepiness, narcolepsy is often associated with cataplexy (a sudden loss of muscle control), sleep paralysis, and hallucinations during the sleep-wake transition.

1. **Hormonal Sleep Disturbances**

Hormonal changes related to menstruation, pregnancy, perimenopause, and menopause can cause significant sleep disturbances in women. During menstruation, for example, some women experience disrupted sleep due to hormonal fluctuations that cause discomfort, pain, or mood changes. Pregnancy can cause frequent awakenings due to physical discomfort, heartburn, and anxiety. During perimenopause and menopause, hot flashes, night sweats, and anxiety can interfere with sleep. These hormonal changes can disrupt circadian rhythms, making it more difficult for women to fall and stay asleep.

1. **Circadian Rhythm Disorders**

Circadian rhythm disorders occur when the body's internal clock, which regulates sleep-wake cycles, is misaligned with the external environment. This misalignment can lead to difficulty falling asleep at the right time, waking up too early, or experiencing daytime fatigue. Women may experience circadian rhythm disorders due to shift work, jet lag, or hormonal changes. Managing circadian rhythms through light exposure, proper sleep hygiene, and lifestyle changes is essential for improving sleep quality.

Tips for Improving Sleep Quality and Establishing a Bedtime Routine

Sleep quality is essential for maintaining good health, managing stress, and enhancing cognitive performance. Establishing a bedtime routine and incorporating sleep-promoting habits can significantly improve sleep hygiene and help women achieve better, more restful sleep.

1. **Create a Consistent Sleep Schedule**

Going to bed and waking up simultaneously daily helps regulate the body's internal clock, promoting a natural sleep-wake rhythm. Women should aim for at least 7-9 hours of sleep each night, depending on their age, health status, and individual needs. Consistency is key, even on weekends, to prevent disruptions to the circadian rhythm.

1. **Optimize the Sleep Environment**

A comfortable and conducive sleep environment is crucial for quality rest. Make the bedroom a peaceful, quiet, and dark space. Use blackout curtains to block out light, and consider using a white noise machine if external sounds are disruptive. Ensure that the mattress, pillows, and bedding are supportive and comfortable. The ideal temperature for sleep is typically calm, around 60-67°F (15-20°C), which can help lower the body's core temperature and promote deeper sleep.

1. **Limit Screen Time Before Bed**

Exposure to blue light from screens (smartphones, tablets, computers, televisions) can interfere with melatonin production, the hormone responsible for regulating sleep. Avoid using screens at least 30-60 minutes before bed to help the body wind down and prepare for sleep. Instead, enjoy relaxing activities such as reading, journaling, or meditating.

1. **Incorporate Relaxation Techniques**

Relaxation techniques such as deep breathing, progressive muscle relaxation, and mindfulness meditation can help calm the mind and body before bed. These techniques reduce stress and promote a sense of calmness that is conducive to sleep. Some women may find yoga or gentle stretching before bed to help release physical tension and prepare for sleep.

1. **Avoid Caffeine and Heavy Meals**

Caffeine is a stimulant that can interfere with sleep if consumed too late in the day. It is recommended to avoid caffeinated beverages (coffee, tea, soda) at least 6 hours before bedtime. Additionally, heavy meals or spicy foods close to bedtime can lead to indigestion or heartburn, making sleeping difficult. opt for a light snack if hunger strikes before bed.

1. **Establish a Bedtime Routine**

A calming pre-sleep routine can signal the brain that it is time to wind down. Establishing a bedtime routine that involves soothing activities such as taking a warm bath, reading, or practicing mindfulness can help improve sleep quality. Over time, this routine can make the body and mind transition into a restful sleep state more easily.

1. **Address Underlying Health Conditions**

If sleep disturbances persist, it may be helpful to consult with a healthcare provider to identify and address underlying health issues, such as hormonal imbalances, sleep apnea, or anxiety disorders. Therapy or medications may sometimes be necessary to treat specific sleep disorders.

1. **Exercise Regularly, But Not Close to Bedtime**

Regular physical activity promotes better sleep by reducing stress anxiety and promoting the release of endorphin.

Chapter 14: Aging Gracefully

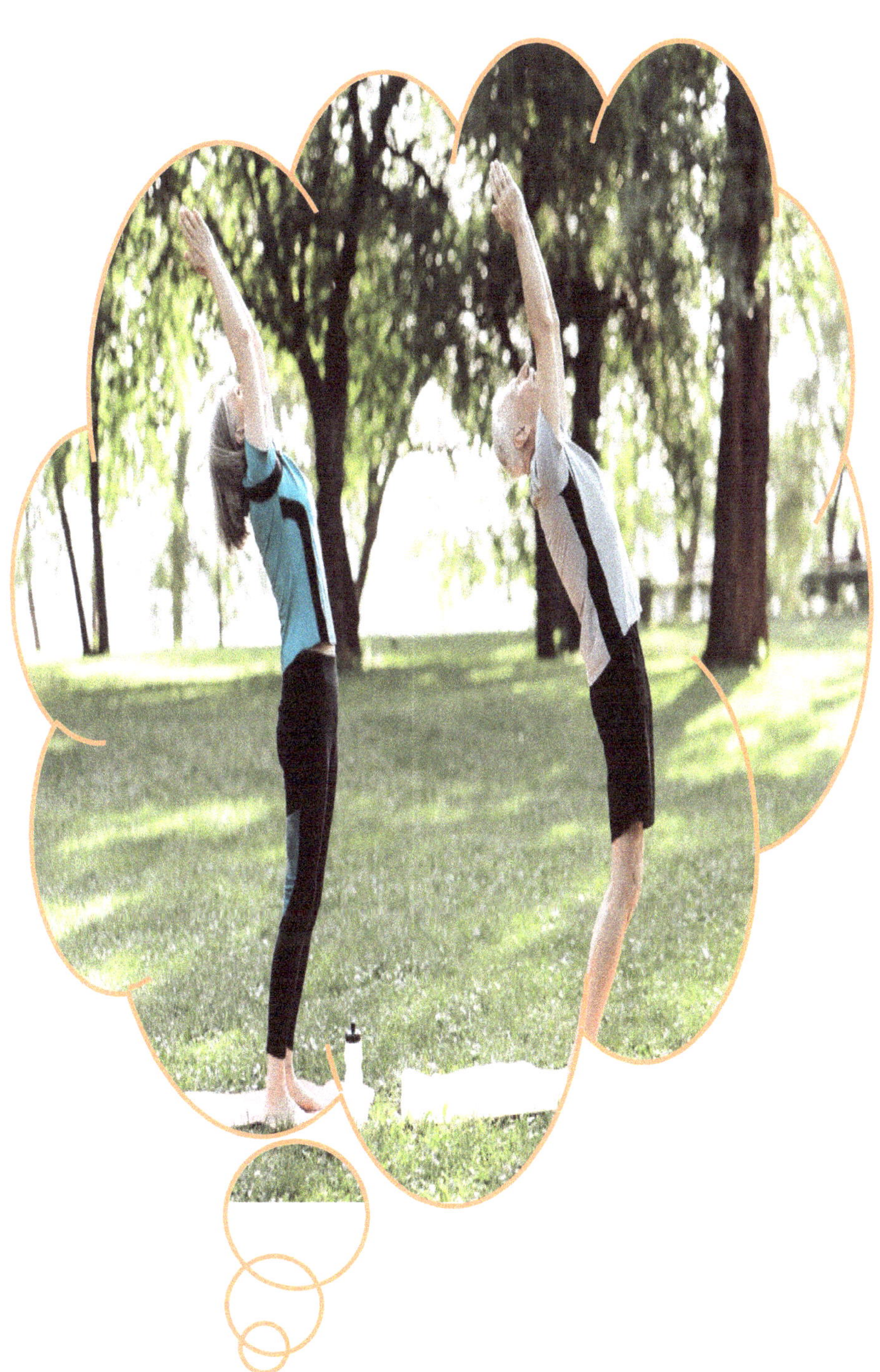

Aging is an inevitable part of life, yet it is often met with anxiety and resistance. However, how we approach aging can significantly affect how we experience the later years of our lives. The concept of aging gracefully is not about denying the passage of time but about embracing it with a mindset that focuses on well-being, vitality, and inner peace. This chapter delves into understanding the aging process and its impact on health, presents strategies for maintaining vitality in older age, and explores the importance of fostering a positive mindset in the face of inevitable changes.

1. Understanding the Aging Process and Its Effects on Health

Aging is a complex and multifaceted process that affects all aspects of the human body. On a biological level, aging refers to the gradual decline of bodily functions and increased susceptibility to diseases and conditions previously rare or non-existent in younger years. A combination of genetic, environmental, and lifestyle factors drives this decline. It is essential to recognize that aging is not a disease but a process that can vary significantly between individuals.

Biological Factors of Aging

Changes primarily drive the biological aging process at the cellular level. Over time, cells accumulate damage from various sources, including oxidative stress, DNA mutations, and wear and tear from repeated cellular divisions. One of the key mechanisms contributing to aging is telomere shortening. Telomeres are protective caps at the ends of chromosomes that shorten each time a cell divides. As telomeres become shorter, the cell loses its ability to divide and function properly, contributing to aging.

Another aspect of aging at the cellular level is mitochondrial dysfunction. Mitochondria, the energy-producing structures within cells, become less efficient with age, reducing overall energy production. This reduction in cellular energy impacts various tissues and organs, including the muscles, brain, and heart.

Physical Changes in the Body

As people age, they experience several physical changes, including:

- **Skin:** Over time, the skin loses elasticity, becomes thinner, and may develop wrinkles. This occurs because the production of collagen and elastin, which provide skin with strength and elasticity, declines.
- **Musculoskeletal System:** Muscle mass and bone density tend to decrease with age. This leads to weaker muscles and more fragile bones, increasing the risk of fractures and falls.
- **Cardiovascular System:** The heart may become less efficient at pumping blood, and blood vessels may stiffen, leading to higher blood pressure and an increased risk of cardiovascular disease.
- **Endocrine System:** Hormonal changes associated with aging can affect metabolism, reproductive health, and energy levels. For

example, estrogen and testosterone levels decline, and insulin sensitivity decreases, which can contribute to conditions like diabetes.

- **Cognitive Function:** Age-related changes in the brain can lead to cognitive decline, including memory loss, slower processing speeds, and difficulty concentrating. However, significant cognitive decline is not an inevitable part of aging and can often be mitigated with proper care and lifestyle choices.

Psychological Changes

As we age, psychological changes can also take place. Seniors may experience emotional shifts related to life transitions, such as retirement, loss of loved ones, or changes in health. These transitions can sometimes lead to feelings of isolation, sadness, or anxiety, mainly if individuals have not developed strong coping mechanisms.

Despite these challenges, many older adults report increased emotional resilience, wisdom, and satisfaction with life. The ability to engage with the world, form meaningful relationships, and maintain a sense of purpose can mitigate the impact of negative emotional states.

1. Strategies for Maintaining Health and Vitality in Older Age

While aging brings inevitable changes, numerous strategies are available to help individuals maintain health, vitality, and independence as they age. These strategies span physical health, mental well-being, and lifestyle choices.

Physical Health

- **Exercise and Physical Activity:** Regular physical activity is one of the most effective ways to maintain health in older age. Exercise can improve cardiovascular health, strengthen bones and muscles, and enhance flexibility and balance, reducing fall risk. Aerobic workouts, such as walking, swimming, or cycling, can boost heart health, while strength training exercises help maintain muscle mass and bone density.
- **Balanced Diet:** Nutrition plays a vital role in healthy aging. Older adults must ensure they consume adequate nutrients, particularly those that tend to decline with age, such as calcium, vitamin D, and B12. A well-balanced diet rich in fruits, vegetables, whole grains, lean proteins, and healthy fats helps support immune function, energy levels, and cognitive health.
- **Hydration:** Dehydration can become a significant concern as people age because the body's ability to retain fluids diminishes. Proper hydration is essential for maintaining energy levels, preventing constipation, and supporting kidney function.
- **Regular Check-ups:** Preventative healthcare, including regular check-ups and screenings, is crucial for identifying potential health issues early. Blood pressure, cholesterol, and glucose levels should be

monitored, and screenings for certain cancers, osteoporosis, and cognitive function should be a part of regular health maintenance.

- **Sleep Hygiene:** As people age, sleep patterns often change, with many older adults experiencing difficulty sleeping. However, maintaining good sleep hygiene can help improve sleep quality. Creating a restful sleep environment, following a consistent sleep schedule, and avoiding stimulants such as caffeine can promote better sleep.

Mental Well-being

- **Cognitive Stimulation:** Keeping the brain active is vital for maintaining mental health. Engaging in mentally stimulating activities like reading, solving puzzles, learning new skills, or playing musical instruments can help preserve memory and cognitive function. Lifelong learning has been shown to protect against cognitive decline and may delay the onset of dementia.
- **Stress Management:** Chronic stress can have a detrimental impact on both physical and mental health. Meditation, mindfulness, yoga, and deep-breathing exercises can help manage stress and improve emotional well-being. These practices can also enhance mental clarity and improve overall mood.
- **Social Connections:** Maintaining strong social networks is associated with better health outcomes in older adults. Social isolation and loneliness can contribute to depression, cognitive decline, and poorer physical health. Engaging in community activities, maintaining friendships, and spending time with family members can positively impact mental health.

Emotional Health

- **Mindfulness and Acceptance:** Embracing aging with a positive attitude involves accepting the changes that come with time. Mindfulness practices promoting self-awareness and acceptance can help individuals adjust to changes in their bodies and lives. Cultivating gratitude for the present moment and focusing on the positive aspects of aging can foster resilience and improve emotional well-being.
- **Purpose and Meaning:** Having a sense of purpose in life is associated with longer life expectancy and better quality of life. This can come from various sources, including hobbies, volunteering, spiritual practices, or family involvement. Maintaining a sense of purpose helps individuals stay motivated, active, and engaged.

1. Embracing Changes and Fostering a Positive Mindset

A positive mindset is the most crucial element of aging gracefully. While it is natural to feel concerned about the changes that come with aging, it is possible to foster a mindset that embraces these changes and focuses on the opportunities that come with them.

Changing Perspectives on Aging

One of the first steps in embracing aging is altering societal perceptions. Many cultures have historically viewed aging negatively, associating it with decline, frailty, and loss. However, a growing movement encourages individuals to redefine aging as a time of growth, opportunity, and wisdom. This shift in perspective can empower people to view aging as a continuation of their journey rather than the end of it.

Building Resilience

Resilience is the ability to bounce back from adversity and maintain mental strength in facing challenges. Developing resilience involves learning to cope with stress, developing problem-solving skills, and staying connected to sources of support. Resilient individuals are better equipped to handle the challenges of aging, such as physical decline, loss of independence, and changing family dynamics.

Fostering Positive Relationships

The relationships we cultivate in our later years are often a source of strength and emotional fulfillment. Maintaining meaningful connections with family members, friends, and community members can provide a buffer against the challenges of aging. These relationships contribute to feelings of belonging and purpose, essential for mental and emotional health.

Accepting Change with Grace

A key aspect of aging gracefully is learning to accept the changes that come with aging. Rather than fighting against these changes, individuals can learn to embrace them as part of the natural flow of life. This involves adjusting expectations, letting go of unrealistic standards, and focusing on what can still be accomplished, enjoyed, and experienced.

Looking Ahead with Optimism

Aging gracefully is about looking forward with optimism rather than focusing on what is lost. It involves setting new goals, trying new activities, and finding joy in the present moment. Optimism and hopefulness can improve physical health, emotional resilience, and overall life satisfaction.

Conclusion

Aging gracefully is about more than just maintaining physical health—it's about embracing the inevitable changes of aging with a positive and open mindset. By understanding the biological, physical, and psychological aspects of aging, individuals can take proactive steps to maintain their health and vitality. Adopting strategies that promote physical, mental, and emotional well-being and foster a positive outlook on life can help individuals navigate the aging process with grace and dignity. Aging is not a loss but an opportunity to live fully with greater wisdom, purpose, and joy.

Chapter 15: Myths and Misconceptions in Women's Health

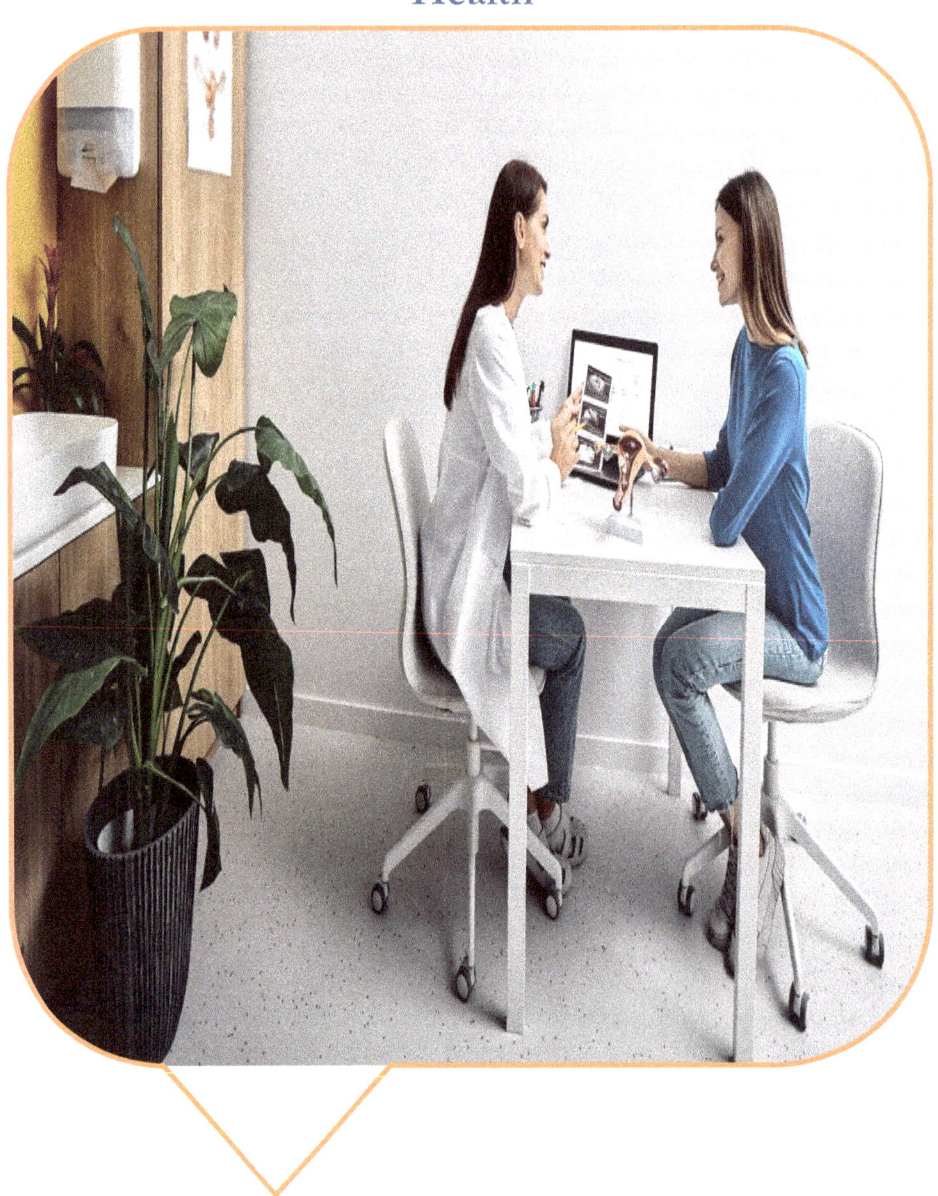

Women's Myths and misconceptions have long clouded women's health, some rooted in cultural beliefs, societal expectations, and even misinformation spread through social media and less reliable sources. This chapter aims to shed light on these myths, debunking them with scientifically backed evidence. Additionally, it emphasizes the importance of critical thinking when evaluating health-related information, as misinformation can often lead to detrimental health outcomes.

1. Common Myths Surrounding Women's Health Issues

1.1 Myth 1: Birth Control Pills Cause Infertility

One of the most pervasive myths is that using birth control pills for extended periods can lead to infertility. This myth stems from misunderstandings about the way hormonal contraceptives work. While hormonal birth control alters a woman's hormonal levels to prevent pregnancy, it does not permanently affect fertility. Once a woman stops taking birth control, her fertility typically returns to normal within a few months.

Evidence: Studies have shown that fertility is usually restored within three months after discontinuation of oral contraceptives. The American College of Obstetricians and Gynecologists (ACOG) affirms that birth control does not have lasting effects on fertility.

1.2 Myth 2: Women Are More Likely to Develop Osteoporosis Than Men

While it's true that women are at a higher risk for osteoporosis, particularly after menopause, this doesn't mean that men are immune to the disease. Osteoporosis is a condition characterized by weakened bones, not exclusive to women.

Evidence: Osteoporosis is a significant health risk for both genders, though women are more likely to experience it due to hormonal changes post-menopause. However, men also have osteoporosis, especially as they age and their testosterone levels decline.

1.3 Myth 3: Menopause Starts at Age 50

While the average age of menopause is 51, it is not a hard and fast rule. The onset of menopause can vary significantly among women, with some experiencing symptoms earlier or later than 50. Early menopause can occur due to various factors, including genetics, autoimmune diseases, or surgical removal of the ovaries.

Evidence: The North American Menopause Society explains that menopause occurs in women between the ages of 40 and 58, but the average age is 51. Genetic factors and lifestyle choices can also affect the timing of menopause.

1.4 Myth 4: Women Should Avoid Exercise During Pregnancy

Another common myth is that women should avoid exercise during pregnancy to prevent harm to the baby. Moderate physical activity during pregnancy can benefit the mother and the baby unless contraindicated by a healthcare provider due to specific medical conditions.

Evidence: According to the American College of Obstetricians and Gynecologists, regular physical activity during pregnancy can reduce the risk of gestational diabetes, improve mood, and help with weight management. Activities like walking, swimming, and prenatal yoga are typically safe for pregnant women.

1.5 Myth 5: You Can't Get Pregnant During Your Period

Many people mistakenly believe that a woman cannot get pregnant during her period. However, sperm can survive in the female reproductive tract for up to five days. If a woman has a short menstrual cycle, she may ovulate shortly after her period, making it possible for sperm to fertilize an egg.

Evidence: Research indicates that the timing of ovulation can vary among women. While it is less likely to become pregnant during menstruation, it is not impossible, particularly for women with irregular cycles.

1. **Debunking Misinformation with Evidence-Based Facts**

2.1 Understanding the Role of Hormones in Women's Health

Many myths surrounding women's health are tied to misconceptions about hormones. For instance, some believe that all hormonal changes in women are inherently problematic or lead to disease, but this is not the case.

Evidence: Hormones naturally fluctuate throughout a woman's life, especially during menstruation, pregnancy, and menopause. This fluctuation can cause temporary symptoms, such as mood swings or fatigue, but these are not inherently harmful. Hormones are crucial in maintaining health, as they regulate metabolism, mood, and bone density.

2.2 The Truth About "Detoxing" Products

There is a significant market for detox products that claim to cleanse the body of toxins and promote weight loss. Many of these products target women, leading to misconceptions about the need for detoxing.

Evidence: The human body has natural detoxification systems, including the liver, kidneys, and digestive system, that effectively eliminate waste. There is little scientific evidence to support the claims of detox products, and some may even cause harm. The U.S. National Institutes of Health (NIH) states that detox diets are unnecessary for healthy individuals.

2.3 The Myth of the "Perfect" Body Image

In a society that often equates beauty with health, many myths revolve around the idea of a "perfect" body. These ideals can contribute to body image issues, such as eating disorders and low self-esteem. The belief that women must look a sure way to be healthy or happy is misleading.

Evidence: Studies have shown that body diversity is normal and that appearance alone cannot accurately determine health. Factors like genetics, physical activity, and mental health are better indicators of overall well-being than body shape or size. The National Eating Disorders Association stresses the importance of accepting one's body as part of overall mental and physical health.

2.4 The "50% of Women Will Get Breast Cancer" Fallacy

Breast cancer is a leading health concern for women, but a common misconception is that 50% of women will develop the disease in their lifetime. This statistic is misleading and overstates the actual risk.

Evidence: According to the American Cancer Society, about 1 in 8 women (12%) will develop breast cancer in their lifetime, not 50%. The lifetime risk is influenced by factors such as genetics, lifestyle, and environmental exposures, and early detection through screening can significantly reduce the risk of death.

2.5 The Myth of "Natural" vs. "Synthetic" Hormones

There is a widespread belief that "natural" hormones (often referred to as bioidentical hormones) are safer and more effective than "synthetic" hormones used in hormone replacement therapy (HRT). This myth has led to confusion and, in some cases, avoidance of medically necessary treatments.

Evidence: Based on a woman's health needs, the FDA has stated that synthetic and bioidentical hormones can be safe and effective when appropriately prescribed. The key factor is not whether the hormone is natural or artificial but the method of administration and dosage that suits the individual.

1. **Importance of Critical Thinking in Health-Related Information**

3.1 The Influence of Media and Social Media on Women's Health Beliefs

The rise of social media has significantly impacted how women receive health information. While it provides access to a wealth of knowledge, it also spreads misinformation that can lead to poor health decisions.

Evidence: Research indicates that health information shared on social media can be misleading, especially from unverified sources. A study published in JAMA found that health information on social media platforms was often inaccurate, which can contribute to dangerous health behaviors.

3.2 How to Evaluate Health Information Critically

Critical thinking involves evaluating health claims' credibility, source, and evidence. Women should question the validity of health advice, especially from unknown or unverified sources, such as social media influencers or websites with no medical expertise.

Evidence: Critical thinking skills can be learned and practiced. The American Medical Association recommends verifying the credentials of health professionals before trusting their advice and seeking peer-reviewed sources when in doubt. Websites like PubMed and government health sites (e.g., the

Centers for Disease Control and Prevention) provide evidence-based information.

3.3 Recognizing the Role of Peer Pressure and Cultural Norms in Health Decisions

Peer pressure and societal norms can strongly influence women's health choices. For instance, women may feel compelled to follow diet trends or undergo unnecessary cosmetic surgeries due to social pressure or media portrayals of ideal beauty standards.

Evidence: Research on body image and societal pressure highlights that external influences can affect women's mental and physical health. Studies suggest that social media plays a significant role in shaping attitudes about body image and health, leading many to pursue harmful practices like extreme dieting or surgery.

3.4 The Importance of Seeking Professional Medical Advice

While the internet and social media offer vast information, women must seek professional medical advice when making health decisions. A healthcare provider, particularly one who understands the unique aspects of women's health, can offer personalized guidance and ensure that health choices are based on sound scientific evidence.

Evidence: According to the World Health Organization (WHO), healthcare providers are critical in ensuring patients receive accurate, up-to-date information and that treatment plans are appropriate to their specific health needs.

Conclusion

The myths and misconceptions surrounding women's health are numerous, but they can be overcome through education, critical thinking, and reliance on evidence-based information. Women must be empowered with knowledge, and society must work to ensure that health information is accurate and accessible. By debunking common myths, addressing misinformation, and encouraging critical thinking, we can improve women's health outcomes and help them make informed decisions about their well-being.

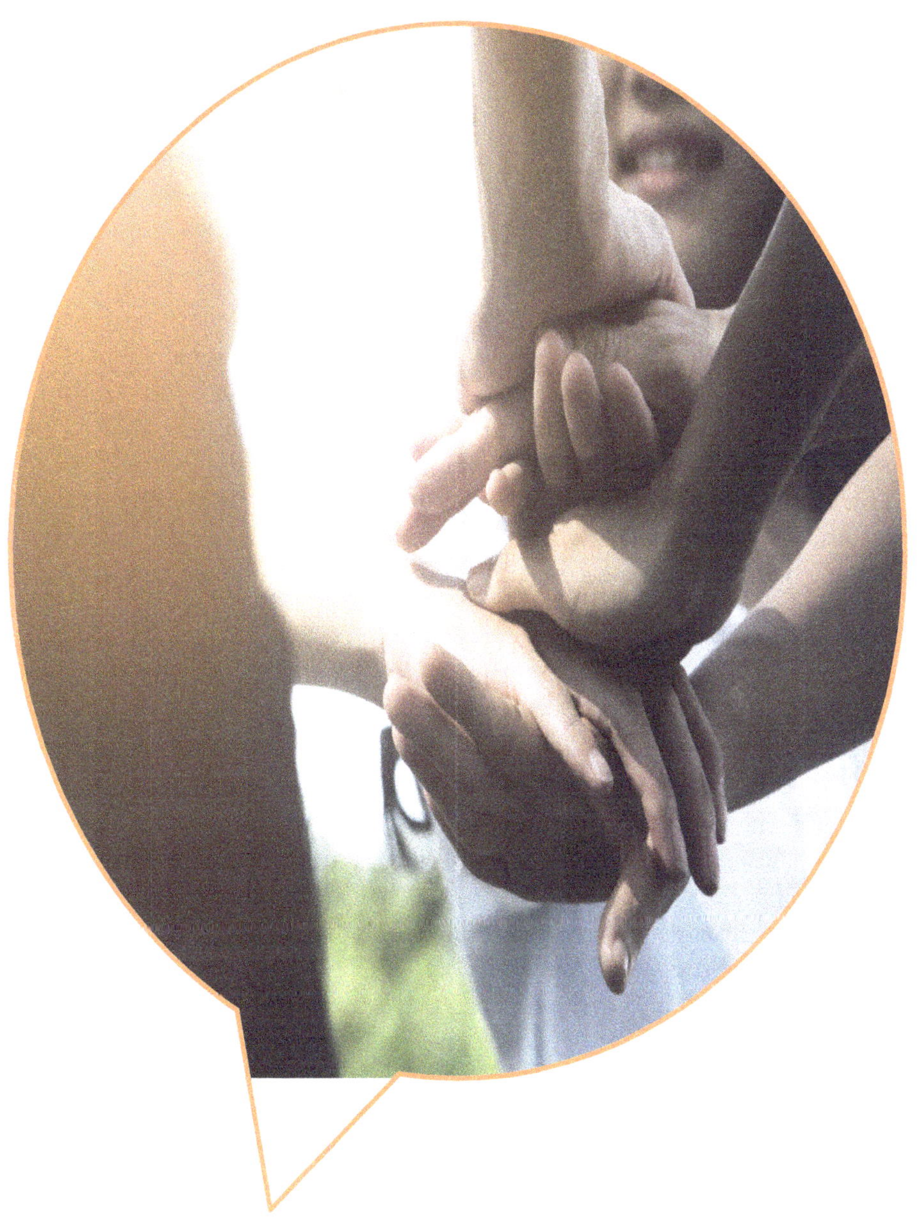

Introduction to Building a Support Network

A support network is essential for emotional well-being, particularly for women, who often juggle various roles and responsibilities. Building and maintaining a robust support system can significantly impact mental, emotional, and physical health. This chapter delves into the role of social support in women's health, how to cultivate meaningful relationships, and resources for finding support groups and communities.

The Role of Social Support in Women's Health

1. Defining Social Support

Social support refers to the psychological and material resources others provide that help individuals cope with stress and adversity. It can take the form of emotional support (e.g., empathy, encouragement), instrumental support (e.g., financial assistance, physical help), informational support (e.g., advice, guidance), and appraisal support (e.g., feedback on decisions). Women, in particular, benefit from a robust support system due to their unique social roles, caregiving responsibilities, and societal expectations.

2. The Impact of Social Support on Women's Physical Health

Research consistently highlights the importance of social support in enhancing women's physical health. Studies show that women with strong social connections are at a lower risk for chronic illnesses, such as heart disease and hypertension. A supportive network improves immune function and enhances recovery outcomes following illness or surgery.

3. Mental and Emotional Health Benefits

Emotional support plays a crucial role in managing mental health challenges such as depression, anxiety, and stress. Women often experience higher rates of anxiety and depression, mainly due to social pressures and caregiving burdens. A solid support network provides a buffer against these mental health struggles by offering a sense of belonging, reducing feelings of isolation, and enhancing emotional resilience.

4. Coping with Stress and Adversity

Women are more likely to experience stress due to the demands placed on them in both their professional and personal lives. A support network helps mitigate stress by allowing individuals to talk, offering practical solutions, and reminding them of their strengths. Support systems are also crucial in times of crisis, such as the death of a loved one, divorce, or serious illness, by providing both emotional and practical assistance.

5. Support and Reproductive Health

In the context of reproductive health, social support can be particularly influential. Women undergoing pregnancy, childbirth, or menopause often experience heightened emotional and physical challenges. Having a trusted support network during these times can reduce feelings of overwhelm, improve mental health, and even enhance physical outcomes (e.g., quicker recovery post-childbirth and better management of menopause symptoms).

How to Cultivate Meaningful Relationships

1. Self-awareness and Identifying Needs

Understanding one's needs is the first step in building a meaningful support network. This involves self-reflection and self-awareness, where women evaluate their emotional, psychological, and physical requirements. Are they seeking emotional support, practical assistance, or a balance? Identifying what is needed from relationships helps focus efforts on forming the most beneficial connections.

2. Building Trust and Vulnerability

Trust is the cornerstone of any meaningful relationship. Women need to open up and be vulnerable to cultivate relationships that provide substantial support. While this can be difficult for many, especially given societal norms around women's emotional labor, allowing oneself to be vulnerable is essential for deepening relationships. Vulnerability leads to stronger emotional bonds, which, in turn, make support more genuine and lasting.

3. Prioritizing Quality Over Quantity

One common misconception is that a large social circle is necessary for a strong support network. However, cultivating a few high-quality, meaningful relationships is far more valuable than having a broad range of acquaintances. Women should focus on nurturing connections where mutual respect, trust, and emotional fulfillment are prioritized over the mere number of people they know.

4. Communicating Needs Clearly

Often, women are socialized to prioritize others' needs over their own. However, to build an effective support network, it is crucial to communicate one's needs clearly and assertively. Whether asking for help with childcare, requesting emotional support during a tough time, or simply seeking a safe space to vent, being open about what is needed from relationships allows others to respond accordingly.

5. Practicing Empathy and Reciprocity

Meaningful relationships are built on empathy and reciprocity. Both parties need to feel supported and valued. Women should invest in their relationships by practicing active listening, offering emotional support when needed, and showing appreciation for the people in their lives. When relationships are reciprocal, they tend to be more sustainable and fulfilling over time.

6. Setting Boundaries

Establishing and maintaining boundaries is a key aspect of cultivating healthy relationships. This helps prevent burnout and ensures that one's emotional and physical energy is preserved for those who genuinely matter. Setting boundaries also communicates respect for oneself and the other party, ensuring that interactions are healthy and supportive, not draining.

7. Overcoming Obstacles in Relationship Building

Building meaningful relationships can be challenging, especially for women with past trauma, trust issues, or conflicting schedules. Women need to approach these obstacles with patience and a growth mindset. Seeking professional guidance, such as therapy or counseling, can help navigate these challenges and foster healthier relationships in the long term.

Resources for Finding Support Groups and Communities

1. Online Support Groups

In today's digital age, finding support has become easier than ever. Online support groups allow women to connect with others facing similar challenges, regardless of geographical location. Websites like Meetup, Facebook groups, and specialized platforms like Reddit or Health Unlocked can connect women with others who share common interests, health challenges, or life experiences.

For example, online groups dedicated to maternal health, mental wellness, or chronic illness can offer shared knowledge and emotional validation. Women can gain practical advice, learn coping strategies, and receive emotional comfort from those who truly understand their struggles.

2. Community-Based Support Groups

In addition to online resources, community-based support groups can be invaluable. Many local community centers, healthcare providers, and nonprofit organizations host support groups tailored to women's health and wellness. These include groups for new mothers, women dealing with chronic illnesses, or support for women undergoing major life transitions.

Organizations such as the YWCA, the Red Cross, or local chapters of organizations like the National Women's Health Network (NWHN) often have resources or can direct women to nearby support groups. Attending in-person meetings can provide a sense of community, allowing for more personal and meaningful connections than digital spaces can often offer.

3. Professional Networks and Therapists

Many women find that working with a therapist or counselor can be an essential step in building a supportive network. Therapists can guide women through the process of cultivating meaningful relationships while also helping to heal past emotional wounds. Additionally, therapists often connect women with support groups tailored to specific challenges, such as grief, trauma, or mental health struggles.

Professional networks for women in various fields, such as women's professional associations, mentorship programs, and advocacy groups, can offer social support in the workplace and help women build supportive relationships that are emotionally and professionally fulfilling.

4. Religious and Spiritual Communities

For many women, religious or spiritual communities provide a crucial source of support. These communities often create a sense of belonging, purpose, and spiritual wellness. Churches, mosques, synagogues, and other religious institutions regularly host support groups or social gatherings that provide emotional support during distress or transition. These spaces also foster deep, trusting relationships based on shared beliefs and values.

5. Support Resources for Specific Life Stages

Support groups and resources are also tailored to specific life stages or experiences. For example, women going through menopause or dealing with infertility can find support in specialized groups that cater to their needs. This focus allows for more targeted advice, understanding, and encouragement. Various healthcare organizations and online platforms offer groups or resources for women navigating these experiences.

6. Local Support Initiatives

Local governments or municipalities often provide support initiatives for women, including assistance with childcare, mental health services, and job training programs. These initiatives create safe spaces for women to connect and share experiences, fostering emotional and practical support within a local context. Women can broaden their support networks by participating in these programs while gaining access to crucial resources.

7. Volunteering and Support Roles

Engaging in volunteer work is another excellent way to build a supportive network. Volunteering for causes that resonate with a woman's values—such as supporting survivors of domestic violence, advocating for women's rights, or working with children—can create bonds with like-minded individuals. These relationships are often rooted in shared purpose and compassion, leading to lasting connections.

Conclusion

Building a strong support network is a cornerstone of women's health and well-being. Social support offers emotional relief during times of stress or crisis and plays a fundamental role in improving physical health, coping with life transitions, and maintaining long-term resilience. Women who cultivate meaningful relationships, communicate their needs and seek out the right resources are better equipped to handle life's challenges. By prioritizing creating supportive, reciprocal, and empathetic relationships, women can foster a network that nurtures their well-being and allows them to thrive in all areas of life.

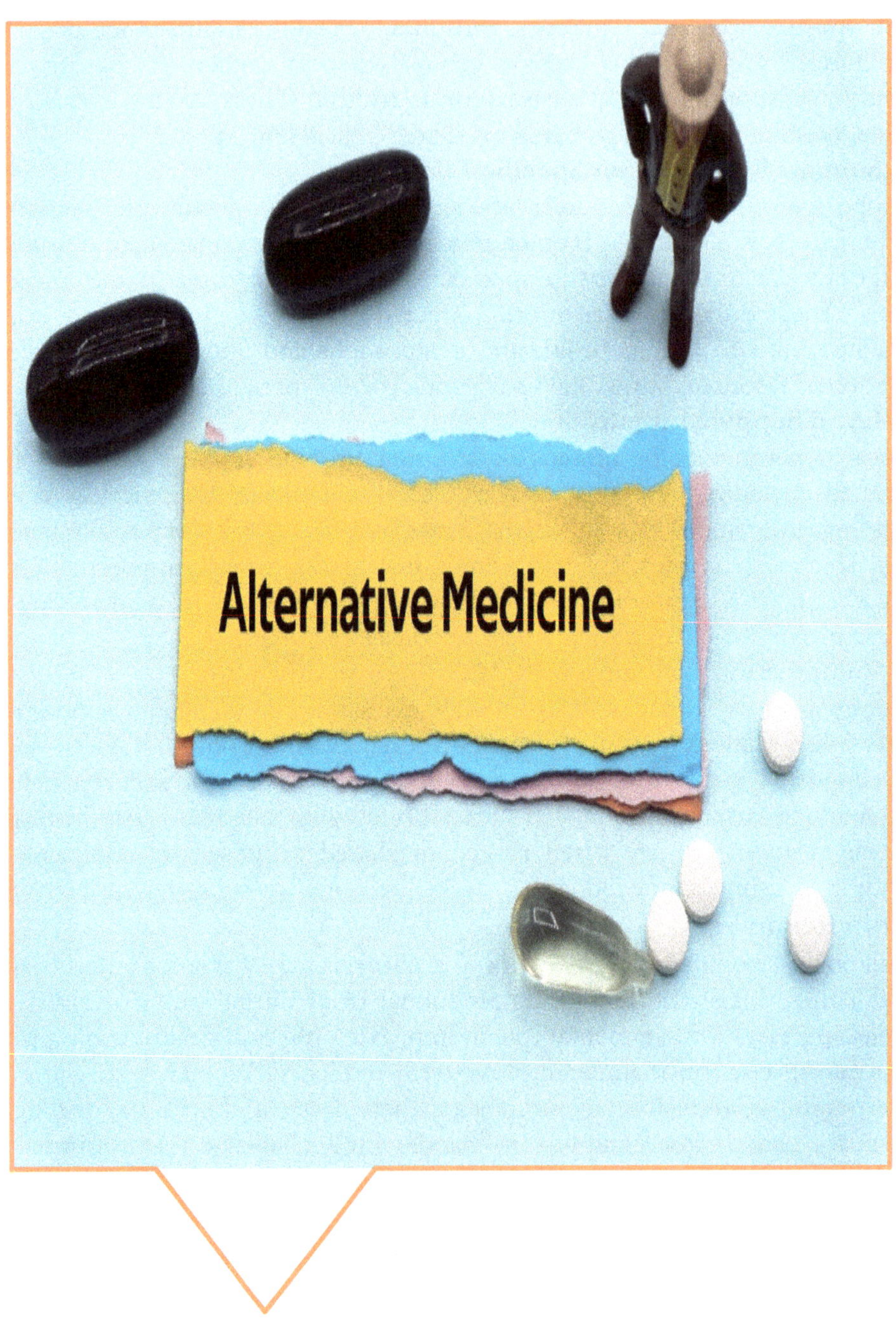
Alternative Medicine

Overview of Integrative Health Approaches (e.g., Acupuncture, Yoga)

Integrative health approaches are a holistic approach to well-being that blends conventional medical treatments with evidence-based complementary practices. These practices aim to treat the whole person—body, mind, and spirit—rather than just addressing symptoms. This chapter will explore some of the most well-known integrative and alternative therapies, including acupuncture, yoga, massage therapy, herbal medicine, and others, to better understand their role in modern health care.

1.1 Defining Integrative Health

Integrative health care refers to a systems-oriented approach that combines the strengths of conventional medical treatment with complementary therapies. Unlike alternative medicine, which stands apart from conventional practices, integrative medicine works alongside traditional medical interventions. The goal is to provide patients with a comprehensive, individualized treatment plan that addresses physical, emotional, mental, and spiritual needs.

1.2 Popular Integrative Health Approaches

- **Acupuncture:** A traditional Chinese medicine (TCM) technique that involves inserting thin needles into specific points on the body to balance energy (Qi) and stimulate healing. Acupuncture effectively manages pain, improves circulation, and promotes well-being.
- **Yoga:** In ancient India, yoga is a physical and philosophical approach to life. The physical practice involves asanas (postures), breathwork (pranayama), and meditation, all fostering mind-body harmony. Yoga has been shown to reduce stress, improve flexibility, and promote emotional balance.
- **Massage Therapy** includes techniques such as Swedish massage, deep tissue massage, and shiatsu. It reduces muscle tension, improves circulation, and promotes relaxation.
- **Herbal Medicine:** The use of plants or plant extracts for medicinal purposes. Herbs like turmeric, echinacea, and ginseng are known for their potential health benefits, ranging from anti-inflammatory properties to immune support.

1.3 Holistic Health and the Mind-Body Connection

A foundational principle in integrative health is the understanding that the mind and body are interconnected. Many therapies above emphasize the importance of balancing emotional, psychological, and physical health. Yoga, for instance, promotes mindfulness, helping individuals become more aware of their thoughts and emotions, which can, in turn, affect their physical health. This mind-body connection is a key component of integrative health approaches.

Benefits and Considerations of Alternative Therapies

While integrative health approaches can benefit many individuals, it is important to consider the advantages and potential challenges of incorporating these therapies into a health journey.

2.1 Benefits of Integrative and Alternative Therapies

- **Personalized Care:** Integrative therapies focus on the individual as a whole. Unlike the "one-size-fits-all" approach sometimes seen in conventional medicine, integrative health practitioners consider a person's lifestyle, diet, emotional state, and other factors when recommending treatment options.
- **Holistic Healing:** These therapies aim to treat the root cause of ailments rather than just alleviating symptoms. For example, acupuncture might help relieve pain, improve energy levels, reduce stress, and enhance sleep quality.
- **Reduction of Side Effects:** Complementary therapies, such as yoga, massage, and herbal medicine, tend to have fewer side effects than pharmaceutical treatments, appealing to those looking for more natural or less invasive alternatives.
- **Stress Reduction:** Many integrative therapies, particularly yoga and acupuncture, help reduce stress levels by activating the body's parasympathetic nervous system (the rest-and-digest response). This can lead to improvements in overall mental health and well-being.
- **Chronic Pain Management:** Acupuncture, massage therapy, and certain forms of yoga are particularly effective for managing chronic pain, especially conditions such as arthritis, back pain, and headaches.
- **Mental Health Benefits:** Yoga and meditation have been shown to reduce symptoms of anxiety and depression. Mindfulness-based practices are also integral to many alternative therapies, offering individuals tools to manage emotional well-being.
- **Improved Quality of Life:** When combined with conventional treatments, integrative health practices can help improve a person's overall quality of life by supporting better physical, emotional, and mental health.

2.2 Considerations and Challenges

While there are numerous benefits to using integrative and alternative therapies, several factors must be considered before incorporating these practices into one's health journey.

- **Lack of Regulation:** Many alternative therapies are less regulated than conventional medical treatments. This lack of regulation can lead to inconsistent standards of care and the potential for harm if practitioners are not adequately trained.

- **Variable Evidence:** While some integrative therapies, like acupuncture and yoga, have significant scientific evidence supporting their efficacy, others may not have as much research backing their claims. It is essential to evaluate the effectiveness of each therapy critically.
- **Potential Interactions:** Some alternative therapies, mainly herbal remedies, may interact with prescription medications, leading to unwanted side effects. Always consult with a healthcare provider before starting any new complementary therapies.
- **Cost and Accessibility:** Integrative therapies may not always be covered by insurance, and access to qualified practitioners may be limited depending on geographic location. In some cases, the costs of ongoing treatments may be prohibitive for some individuals.
- **Misuse of Therapies:** As with any form of health care, alternative therapies should not be used as a replacement for proven conventional treatments, especially in the case of severe medical conditions like cancer, heart disease, or diabetes. They should be viewed as complementary rather than a substitute for conventional medicine.
- **Psychological Impact:** In some cases, individuals may develop a psychological dependency on alternative therapies, seeking them out for problems that may be better addressed through traditional medical interventions or psychological counseling.

How to Incorporate These Practices into Your Health Journey

Integrating alternative therapies into your health journey requires a thoughtful, personalized approach. Below are some practical steps for safely and effectively incorporating these therapies into your lifestyle.

3.1 Step 1: Consult with a Healthcare Professional

Before starting any integrative or alternative therapy, discussing it with your primary healthcare provider is essential. Your doctor can help you determine whether the treatment is appropriate for your health needs and guide you on any potential risks or interactions with existing treatments.

For example, if you are taking medication for high blood pressure, your doctor may advise caution before starting yoga or acupuncture, as these therapies can influence your blood pressure.

3.2 Step 2: Choose the Right Therapy for Your Needs

Different therapies work for other individuals and health conditions. Understanding what each treatment offers and selecting the one that aligns with your specific health goals is essential.

- **Acupuncture** might be appropriate if you're seeking pain relief or are looking for a natural treatment for chronic conditions like migraines or joint pain.

- **Yoga** could be an excellent choice if you're looking to reduce stress, increase flexibility, or improve your mental health.
- **Massage therapy** is great for muscle tension, stress relief, and promoting relaxation.

3.3 Step 3: Start Slowly and Monitor Progress

It is wise to ease into the practice when starting an alternative therapy. For example, begin with a few yoga classes per week or try acupuncture sessions spaced a week apart. Pay close attention to how your body responds and adjust accordingly. Track any changes in symptoms, emotional states, or overall health to evaluate whether the therapy benefits you.

3.4 Step 4: Incorporate Practices into Your Daily Routine

Integrative therapies are most effective when they are part of a consistent, long-term wellness routine. For example, incorporating a short yoga or meditation practice each morning can help set a positive tone for the day, while acupuncture sessions every few weeks may help maintain a balanced state of health. Consistency is key to reaping the full benefits of these therapies.

3.5 Step 5: Be Open to Modifying Your Approach

As you progress on your health journey, be open to modifying your approach. You may find that specific therapies work better for you than others, or you may need to combine different methods to achieve your desired results. For example, acupuncture may alleviate your pain, but you might find that yoga provides additional emotional balance and energy.

3.6 Step 6: Educate Yourself and Stay Informed

Keep yourself informed about new developments and research regarding integrative therapies. Reading scientific studies, talking to practitioners, and engaging with support groups can help you stay up-to-date and make informed decisions about the treatments you're using.

Conclusion

Integrative and alternative therapies offer valuable tools for enhancing overall health and well-being. From acupuncture and yoga to herbal medicine and massage therapy, these approaches provide a holistic framework for treating the whole person. While they can be highly beneficial, it is essential to approach them with a thoughtful, informed mindset and consult with healthcare professionals to ensure safety and efficacy. By carefully incorporating these practices into your health journey, you can take a proactive, empowered role in your wellness and create a balanced, sustainable path toward optimal health.

Chapter 18: The Role of Technology in Health Management

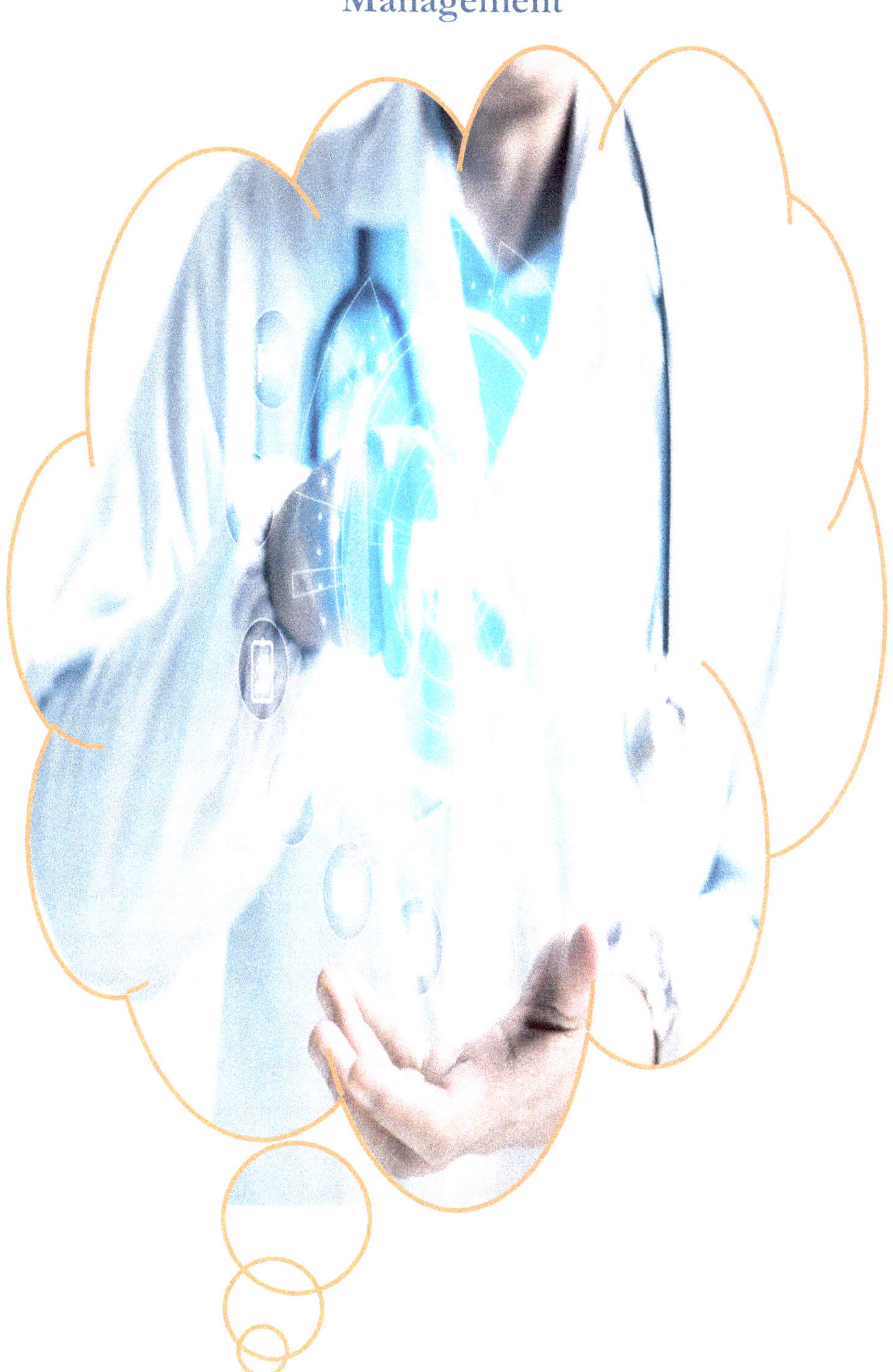

Introduction

Technology has revolutionized the healthcare landscape, transforming how individuals manage their health and access medical services. In recent years, digital health tools, telemedicine, and online resources have become essential to everyday healthcare. The increased integration of technology into health management offers enhanced convenience, accessibility, and personalized care for individuals. This chapter delves into how these technological advancements shape health management, mainly focusing on health apps, wearable technology, telehealth, and reputable online resources.

Utilizing Health Apps and Wearable Technology

1. **Introduction to Health Apps and Wearable Technology**

Health apps and wearable technologies have seen significant growth in recent years. These tools help individuals monitor their health status in real-time, track physical activity, and manage chronic conditions such as diabetes, heart disease, and mental health issues. Health apps can be installed on smartphones, while wearable technologies—such as smartwatches, fitness trackers, and other biometric sensors—are designed to be worn throughout the day to collect data continuously.

1. **Popular Health Apps and Wearable Devices**

Countless health apps are available, each targeting different aspects of health management. Some examples include:

- **MyFitnessPal:** A popular app for tracking diet and exercise.
- **Headspace and Calm:** Apps designed for mental health and mindfulness.
- **Fitbit and Apple Watch:** Wearable devices that monitor physical activity, sleep patterns, heart rate, etc.
- **Glucose monitors for diabetes management** (e.g., Dexcom).

Wearables, like smartwatches, integrate seamlessly with smartphones and can track everything from daily steps to more advanced metrics like blood oxygen levels, ECG readings, and stress levels. These devices can help individuals take proactive steps toward their health, making them more informed about their body's condition.

1. **Benefits of Health Apps and Wearable Technology**

- **Real-time Monitoring:** Constant monitoring helps individuals monitor their health metrics, which is particularly beneficial for managing chronic conditions.
- **Personalized Health Insights:** These technologies collect data over time and can generate customized insights, such as daily activity goals or dietary recommendations based on individual data.
- **Enhanced Engagement:** Health apps and wearables encourage users to engage more with their health by setting reminders and offering motivational feedback.

- **Remote Monitoring:** Healthcare providers can remotely monitor patients with chronic illnesses or those undergoing rehabilitation, reducing the need for frequent in-person visits.

1. **The Role of Wearable Technology in Disease Prevention**

Wearable devices can identify early warning signs of health problems, enabling users to make informed decisions about their health. For instance:

- **Heart Disease Prevention:** Devices that track heart rate variability and irregularities can detect potential cardiac problems.
- **Chronic Disease Management:** Continuous monitoring of glucose levels in diabetics or blood pressure for those at risk of hypertension allows for real-time intervention and better disease management.

1. **Challenges and Considerations**

Despite the numerous benefits, the use of health apps and wearable technology comes with challenges:

- **Data Privacy:** The collection of sensitive health data raises concerns about user privacy and the security of health information.
- **Accuracy of Data:** Some health apps and wearables may only sometimes be entirely accurate, leading to incorrect conclusions and potential risks if users make decisions based on unreliable data.
- **Digital Divide:** Only some have access to the internet or the technology required to use these tools, creating inequalities in health management.

Telehealth and Its Benefits for Women

1. **Overview of Telehealth**

Telehealth uses telecommunications technology, such as video calls, phone consultations, and mobile health apps, to deliver healthcare services remotely. This has been a game-changer, especially for people living in rural areas or individuals with mobility or transportation challenges. Telehealth has seen significant expansion during the COVID-19 pandemic and is a viable option for a wide range of healthcare services.

1. **Telehealth for Women's Health**

Telehealth offers unique advantages for women in managing their health. Women, particularly those in rural or underserved areas, can benefit significantly from remote consultations in areas such as:

- **Prenatal and Postnatal Care:** Women expecting children can access regular check-ups and consultations with healthcare providers without the need to travel long distances.
- **Mental Health Services:** Women experience mental health challenges, including postpartum depression and anxiety disorders, that can be addressed through virtual therapy sessions, making mental health care more accessible.

- **Reproductive Health:** Telehealth allows women to consult gynecologists, obstetricians, and other specialists remotely for contraception advice, menstrual cycle management, and other reproductive health needs.
- **Breast and Cervical Cancer Screenings:** Women can discuss screening results, preventive measures, and treatment options with their healthcare providers through virtual visits, ensuring ongoing care without disruptions.

1. **Benefits of Telehealth for Women**

- **Convenience and Accessibility:** Women with busy schedules—especially those balancing family and work commitments—can access healthcare services from the comfort of their homes, making it easier to manage appointments.
- **Reduced Stigma and Increased Comfort:** Some women may feel more comfortable discussing sensitive issues, such as reproductive health, sexual health, and mental health concerns, in a private telehealth setting rather than in a clinical environment.
- **Chronic Disease Management:** Women managing chronic illnesses, such as diabetes or hypertension, can regularly consult with healthcare professionals, receive medication refills, and monitor their condition remotely.
- **Increased Health Literacy:** Telehealth allows women to engage more actively with their healthcare providers and access educational resources related to their health.

1. **Challenges in Telehealth for Women**

- **Access to Technology:** Like other telemedicine solutions, the availability of high-speed internet and appropriate devices is critical. Women in low-income or rural areas may need help accessing telehealth services.
- **Quality of Care:** While telehealth is effective for many consultations, it may not suit specific examinations requiring in-person visits, such as physical exams or diagnostic procedures.
- **Security and Privacy Concerns:** Virtual healthcare poses challenges in ensuring the privacy of sensitive health information during consultations.

1. **The Future of Telehealth for Women**

With technological advancements and increasing investment in telemedicine infrastructure, the future of telehealth for women looks promising. Integrating AI-driven diagnostics, secure online prescriptions, and enhanced virtual consultations can offer more personalized care. Furthermore, telehealth platforms focusing specifically on women's health needs will likely become more prevalent, allowing for tailored services.

Staying Informed Through Reputable Online Resources

1. **Importance of Reliable Health Information**

With the rapid proliferation of information on the internet, individuals must discern reliable health resources from misinformation. The rise of social media and self-diagnosis platforms has contributed to a significant amount of misinformation about health issues, which can be harmful.

1. **Trusted Sources for Health Information**

Several reputable online platforms provide accurate and evidence-based health information:

- **Government Health Websites (e.g., CDC, WHO):** These platforms offer trustworthy information on health trends, preventive measures, and updates on global health concerns.

- **Non-profit Organizations:** Websites like the American Heart Association, American Diabetes Association, and National Institutes of Health provide reliable information for specific conditions and health advice.

- **Academic and Medical Journals:** Online platforms such as PubMed, the Lancet, and JAMA provide access to peer-reviewed articles and clinical research findings.

1. **Evaluating the Credibility of Online Resources**

Users need to be vigilant when evaluating online health information. Factors to consider include:

- **Authorship:** Information should be written by healthcare professionals or credible organizations with expertise in the subject matter.

- **Evidence-Based:** Information should be supported by scientific research or expert consensus.

- **Transparency:** Reputable websites disclose their sources of funding and conflict of interest.

- **Up-to-date Information:** Health information evolves quickly; therefore, it is essential to consult recent sources.

1. **The Role of Social Media in Health Management**

Social media platforms like Twitter, Instagram, and Facebook are increasingly used for health communication, though they also present challenges. Reputable health organizations and healthcare professionals use social media to educate the public and raise awareness about health issues. However, misinformation can quickly spread on these platforms, making it crucial for individuals to rely on credible voices.

1. **Online Health Communities and Support Groups**

Online health communities, such as forums and virtual support groups, allow individuals to share experiences and seek advice from others facing similar health issues. Though valuable, these communities should be used cautiously, as they are not always a substitute for professional medical advice.

Conclusion

Technology undeniably plays a crucial role in transforming health management, from wearable devices that help track personal health metrics to telehealth services that make healthcare more accessible. For women, these innovations offer opportunities to enhance their health management, reduce barriers to care, and stay informed through reputable online resources. However, these advancements come with challenges, including data privacy concerns, the need for reliable resources, and the digital divide. As healthcare continues to evolve, technology integration promises to improve the quality, accessibility, and efficiency of health services globally.

Chapter 19: Empowering Yourself Through Education

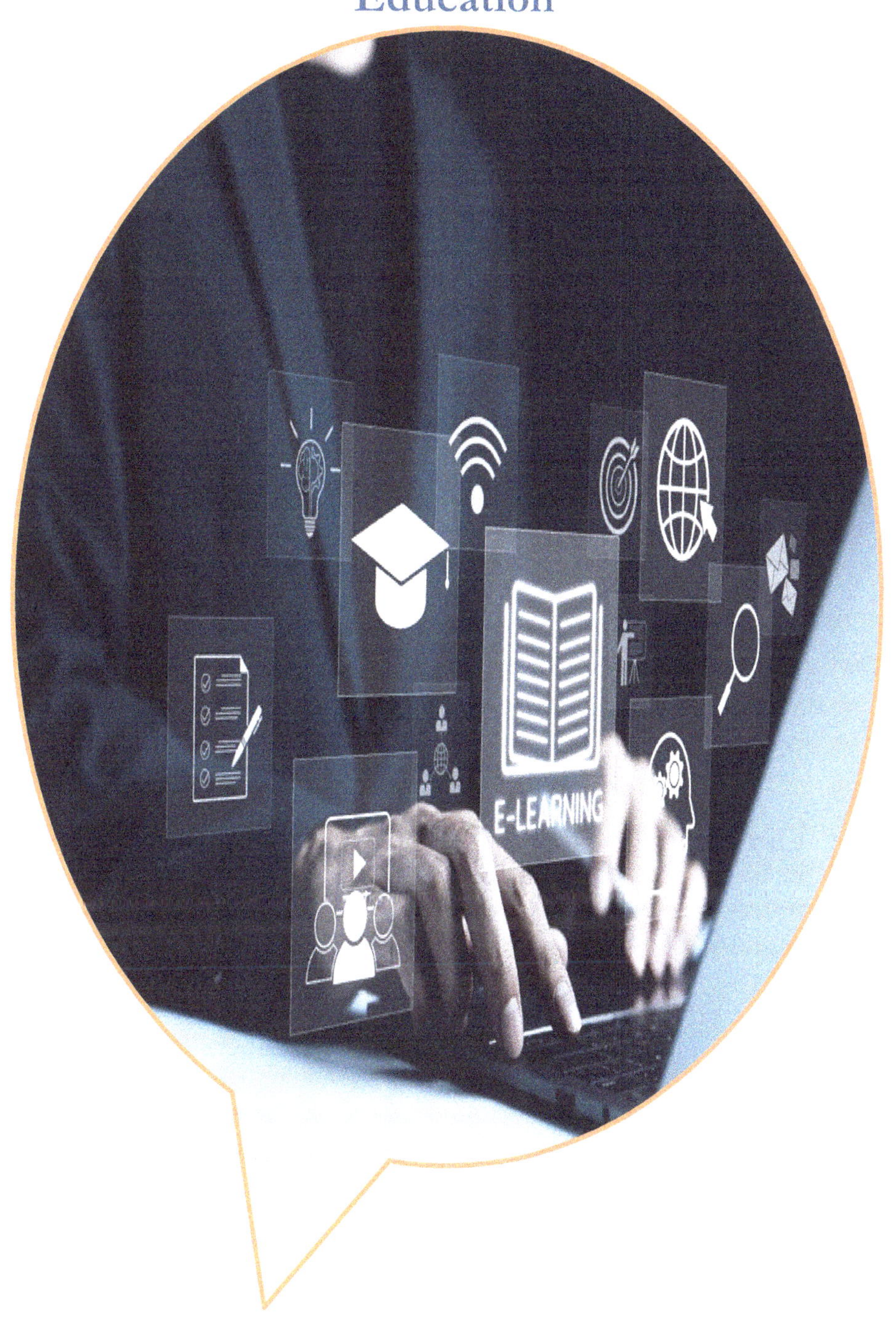

Introduction

Education is the cornerstone of personal empowerment. The more informed we are about our health, the better equipped we are to make sound decisions for ourselves and those around us. Empowerment through education is not limited to gaining knowledge in formal settings; it also extends to learning from various other resources, such as books, websites, workshops, and community-based initiatives. This chapter delves into how education can be a tool for taking charge of your health, how you can continue learning throughout your life, and the importance of advocating for better health education within your community.

Importance of Being Informed About Your Health

Health literacy, the ability to obtain, process, and understand basic health information, is a fundamental aspect of personal empowerment. The more you know about your health, the better decisions you can make to improve your overall well-being. Informed health decisions can prevent unnecessary diseases, reduce medical costs, and improve quality of life.

1. **Making Informed Decisions**

When well-educated about their health, individuals are better able to make decisions that positively impact their well-being. This can include:

- **Understanding Health Risks**: Knowing personal health risks (e.g., genetic predispositions and lifestyle factors like diet and exercise) can help mitigate potential health problems. Early awareness can lead to preventive measures like regular screenings or lifestyle modifications.
- **Navigating the Healthcare System**: By learning more about medical terms, conditions, and treatments, you can better communicate with healthcare providers. This also includes understanding the different healthcare options available, such as traditional medical care, alternative therapies, and holistic approaches.
- **Managing Chronic Conditions**: Understanding chronic conditions in depth can lead to better self-management, fewer complications, and a more active role in treatment decisions for people with them.

1. **Reducing Health Inequalities**

Health education helps bridge gaps in healthcare access, especially in underserved or marginalized communities. Accessing, interpreting, and acting on health information is essential for preventing diseases and improving health outcomes. By empowering individuals to take control of their health, education can reduce disparities in health outcomes based on socioeconomic status, race, or geographic location.

1. **Preventive Health Practices**

A significant aspect of health empowerment through education is the focus on prevention. By understanding the importance of regular checkups, healthy nutrition, physical activity, and mental health care, individuals can avoid more serious illnesses in the future. Knowledge about lifestyle choices such as smoking cessation, reducing alcohol consumption, and stress management can dramatically improve long-term health outcomes.

1. **Mental Health Awareness**

Physical health is only part of the equation; mental health is just as important. Informed individuals are more likely to seek help when experiencing mental health issues, leading to early intervention and better outcomes. Learning about the signs of depression, anxiety, and other mental health conditions is crucial in fostering a healthier society.

Resources for Continued Learning

Lifelong learning is essential in today's rapidly evolving world. Like all knowledge, health knowledge continues to expand as new research emerges. Fortunately, numerous resources are available for continued learning in the field of health and wellness.

1. **Books**

Books remain one of the most reliable sources of in-depth health information. They offer comprehensive insights into various aspects of health, from nutrition and exercise to mental well-being and disease prevention.

- **Health and Wellness Books**: Authors like Dr. Andrew Weil and Dr. Deepak Chopra have popularized the concept of integrative health, offering valuable perspectives on combining traditional and alternative medicine.
- **Medical Textbooks**: For more specific or scientific insights, medical textbooks can provide a more profound understanding of medical conditions, treatments, and healthcare practices.
- **Self-Help and Mental Health Books**: Authors like Brené Brown, Mark Williams, and David Burns offer tools and techniques for enhancing mental health, overcoming anxiety, and developing emotional resilience.

1. **Websites**

In today's digital age, the internet is a vast resource for learning. Many reputable websites offer accurate, evidence-based health information, which can help users stay informed and take proactive steps toward their health.

- **WebMD**: Provides accessible information about symptoms, conditions, treatments, and general health tips.
- **Mayo Clinic**: Known for its reliable, research-backed health content, Mayo Clinic offers in-depth articles on medical conditions and wellness.
- **National Institutes of Health (NIH)**: Offers a comprehensive library of research studies, resources, and publications on various health topics.

- **World Health Organization (WHO)**: A global leader in public health education, WHO's website offers valuable resources on everything from pandemic preparedness to nutrition and mental health.
- **Health Blogs**: Many health experts maintain blogs sharing the latest research, tips, and advice. Some well-known health bloggers include Dr. Mark Hyman (functional medicine) and Dr. Michael Greger (nutrition and lifestyle).

1. **Online Courses and Webinars**

- **Coursera**: Offers many online courses in health-related fields, many from top universities.
- **EdX**: Another platform for university-level courses on health, medicine, and public health topics.
- **TED Talks**: While not formal courses, TED Talks offer thought-provoking presentations on health topics from leading experts.
- **Webinars**: Many health organizations and professionals offer live and recorded webinars on mental health, nutrition, exercise, and disease prevention. These webinars are often free and open to anyone interested.

1. **Workshops and Seminars**

Attending in-person or virtual workshops and seminars can provide hands-on, interactive experiences that enhance your learning. Topics covered may include everything from mindfulness and stress reduction techniques to specific medical treatments and therapeutic practices.

- **Local Health Fairs**: Often held in communities or schools, health fairs provide opportunities to interact with health professionals, ask questions, and learn about the latest health trends.
- **Workshops on Nutrition and Exercise**: These workshops focus on practical tips for adopting healthier lifestyles and can include cooking demonstrations, fitness routines, or mindfulness practices.
- **Support Groups**: Many support groups for chronic health conditions provide an opportunity to learn from others who share similar experiences. These groups often offer educational resources, emotional support, and information about self-care.

1. **Podcasts and Audiobooks**

For those with busy schedules, podcasts and audiobooks can be an excellent alternative to reading. Whether commuting, exercising, or doing household chores, you can continue to educate yourself on health topics during these moments.

- **Podcasts**: Many health professionals and enthusiasts host podcasts covering wellness, fitness, mental health, and healthcare systems.

Notable podcasts include "The Model Health Show" and "Found My Fitness."

- **Audiobooks**: Platforms like Audible provide access to a vast library of health-related audiobooks covering scientific information and personal health journeys.

Encouraging Advocacy and Education in Your Community

As individuals become more educated about their health, they often feel compelled to help others in their communities. Advocating for better health education and resources is a way to amplify the impact of personal empowerment and promote well-being on a larger scale.

1. **Health Education Programs**

One of the most impactful ways to advocate for health education is to create or support health education programs within your community. These programs might focus on:

- **Prevention and Healthy Living**: Teaching people about the importance of healthy habits such as exercise, nutrition, and regular checkups.

- **Mental Health Awareness**: Many communities still lack a basic understanding of mental health. Workshops or seminars focusing on mental health education can help reduce stigma and encourage people to seek help when needed.

- **Chronic Disease Management**: In communities where chronic diseases like diabetes, hypertension, or asthma are prevalent, education programs can empower individuals better to manage their conditions through lifestyle changes and medical adherence.

1. **Volunteer Work**

Volunteering with local health organizations, clinics, or hospitals can be a great way to contribute to health education in your community directly. You can help distribute educational materials, assist in free screening programs, or organize workshops and health fairs.

1. **Partnering with Local Schools**

Schools are a critical space for promoting health education. Partnering with local schools to provide nutrition, exercise, and mental health workshops can lay the foundation for lifelong healthy habits. Students educated about health early on are more likely to carry those lessons into adulthood and pass them on to their families.

1. **Social Media and Online Advocacy**

With the rise of social media, advocating for health education has become easier and more widespread. Through platforms like Facebook, Instagram, Twitter, and TikTok, individuals and organizations can raise awareness about health issues and share valuable information. These platforms can be used to:

- Share accurate health information
- Promote health events and initiatives
- Encourage healthy lifestyle changes
- Foster online communities of support and encouragement

1. **Government and Policy Advocacy**

On a broader scale, advocating for policies that promote health education is crucial. This could involve lobbying for:

- The inclusion of health education in school curricula
- Better access to healthcare resources for underserved communities
- Policies that promote healthier food options in schools and workplaces
- National or local health awareness campaigns

Conclusion

Empowering yourself through education is not just about accumulating facts; it's about transforming your life and community through the knowledge you acquire. The more informed you are about your health, the more control you have over your physical and mental well-being. By utilizing books, websites, workshops, and other learning resources, you can continue to build your health knowledge throughout your life. Furthermore, by advocating for health education and promoting wellness within your community, you can create

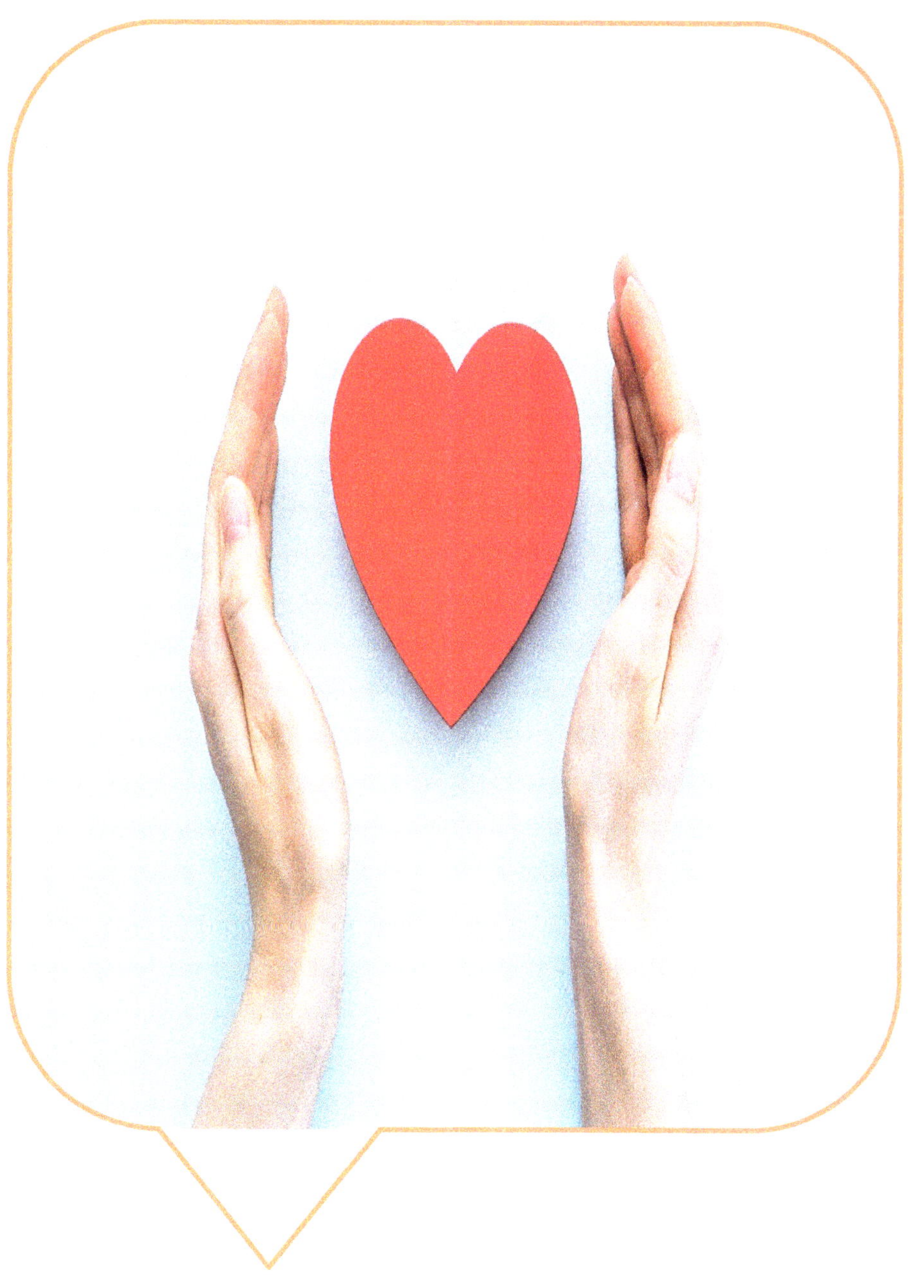

1.   **Recap of Key Themes and Takeaways from the Book**

In the concluding chapter of this book, it's essential to reflect on and summarize the key messages woven throughout the previous chapters. This recap serves not only to reinforce the knowledge gained but also to inspire action as the reader embarks on their health journey.

1.1 Empowerment through Knowledge and Awareness

One of the central themes of this book is the idea that knowledge is power. The book explores various health concepts, from nutrition and fitness to mental well-being and emotional health, and encourages the reader to become fully informed. With knowledge in hand, individuals can make informed choices about their health rather than relying on external authorities or quick-fix solutions.

The message here is clear: you can make decisions affecting your health. Whether you've learned how to fuel your body correctly, understand the importance of regular exercise, or manage stress, the knowledge you've acquired equips you to take charge of your health.

1.2 The Importance of Holistic Health

This book emphasizes a holistic view of health, meaning that it's not just about eating well or exercising. It's about achieving balance across all aspects of life. This includes mental, emotional, and spiritual health, as well as physical well-being. By fostering a sense of balance, individuals can experience a more fulfilling life. Wellness is multifaceted, and to truly take charge of your health, it's important to consider the total picture of your well-being.

1.3 Building Consistency and Habits

Another recurring theme in the book has been the importance of creating sustainable habits. Health is not about short bursts of intense effort followed by periods of neglect; it's about building consistency. The strategies outlined in earlier chapters, such as forming healthy habits, setting realistic goals, and overcoming obstacles, are all part of a larger framework designed to help readers create lasting change.

This section reminds us that small, consistent changes compound over time to create significant long-term results. Health is not a destination but a continuous journey.

1.4 The Role of Mindset in Health and Wellness

A crucial takeaway from this book is the influence of mindset on one's health journey. Maintaining a growth mindset where setbacks are viewed as opportunities for learning rather than failures can significantly affect how one approaches challenges. This positive mindset is essential for overcoming the inevitable hurdles in any health journey and maintaining motivation when things get complicated.

1.5 The Power of Community and Support

While health can often feel like a solitary pursuit, this book has also highlighted the importance of community and support. Whether it's from friends, family, health professionals, or online communities, the support of others can provide encouragement, motivation, and accountability. Surrounding yourself with people who share your health goals can help you stay focused and committed.

1.6 A Lifetime Commitment to Health

Lastly, the book reinforces that health is not a temporary pursuit but a lifelong commitment. There will be ups and downs, but by continually adapting to your body's needs and responding to life's changes, you can maintain a path toward wellness. In this final chapter, the reader is encouraged to focus on health as a short-term goal and lifelong priority.

1. **Creating a Personalized Health Action Plan**

Now that the foundational health and wellness themes have been laid out, it's time to move from theory to action. This focuses This section focuses on helping the reader create a practical, personalized plan that will guide them toward their health goals.

2.1 Understanding Your Unique Health Needs

Before embarking on a health plan, it's essential to take a personalized approach. Every individual has unique health needs based on age, gender, genetics, lifestyle, and existing health conditions. A cookie-cutter approach to health only works for some, so assessing your needs and designing a plan that works for you is essential.

Start by evaluating your current health. This includes:

- **Physical Health:** How do you feel physically? Are there any specific health issues that need addressing, such as weight management, mobility, or chronic conditions like hypertension or diabetes?
- **Mental Health:** Assess your emotional well-being. Do you deal with stress or anxiety regularly? Are you experiencing burnout or burnout-related symptoms?
- **Lifestyle Factors:** Consider your daily routine. Do you get enough sleep, exercise regularly, and eat nutritious foods? How much time do you devote to self-care and relaxation?

2.2 Setting Realistic and Achievable Goals

Goal-setting is crucial for creating a personalized health action plan. However, goals should be realistic, measurable, and achievable. The SMART (Specific, Measurable, Achievable, Relevant, Time-bound) framework is excellent for breaking down larger goals into more minor, manageable actions.

- **Short-term goals** include drinking more water daily, cutting back on sugar, or committing to three days of exercise per week.

- **Long-term Goals:** These could focus on more significant outcomes, such as losing a set amount of weight, reducing cholesterol, or improving mental health through meditation and mindfulness practices.

2.3 Identifying Key Health Pillars

Based on the individual's needs, the next step is to focus on specific areas of health. These pillars could include:

- **Nutrition and Diet:** Tailor a balanced eating plan that provides the necessary nutrients while aligning with your goals. Consider incorporating whole foods, lean proteins, healthy fats, and many fruits and vegetables.
- **Exercise and Physical Activity:** Based on your fitness level, create a program that includes a variety of exercises, such as cardiovascular activities, strength training, flexibility exercises, and rest days.
- **Mental and Emotional Health:** Include meditation, mindfulness, journaling, therapy, or other emotional wellness strategies to help manage stress and enhance mental clarity.
- **Sleep Hygiene:** Good sleep is the foundation of overall well-being. Include strategies for improving sleep quality, such as establishing a regular sleep schedule, limiting screen time before bed, and creating a calming bedtime routine.
- **Social and Community Support:** Ensure that a support system is in place, whether it's family, friends, or a fitness community, to help maintain motivation and accountability.

2.4 Building Consistency and Accountability

Consistency is key in the pursuit of health. Your health action plan should include strategies for staying on track, even when motivation wanes. These could involve setting reminders, tracking progress with journaling or apps, or regularly reassessing goals.

Accountability can also be a game-changer. This can come from a workout buddy, a mentor, a health coach, or even social media support groups. Regular check-ins, even informal ones, can help keep you motivated and ensure you stick to your plan.

2.5 Flexibility and Adaptability

It's crucial to acknowledge that life and your health journey are not static. Health plans should be dynamic, with room for adjustments as needed. This could mean changing your diet based on how your body responds, modifying your exercise routine when life gets busy, or seeking new mental health strategies if your emotional needs change.

Life events such as moving, starting a new job, or dealing with personal challenges may require alterations to your plan. The key is to adapt and keep going.

1. **Encouragement to Embrace the Journey of Health and Wellness**

Finally, as the reader approaches the end of this book, it's essential to leave them with a sense of encouragement and motivation to continue the health journey.

3.1 Health is a Lifelong Journey

Taking charge of your health is not about reaching a singular goal but about continual improvement. Embrace the journey, knowing that every step forward is progress. It's normal to experience setbacks or plateaus, but persistence matters.

3.2 Celebrate Progress, Not Perfection

Health is not about achieving perfection but about progress. Celebrate small wins, whether a new personal best in the gym, eating a nutritious meal, or feeling more energized throughout the day. Acknowledge and appreciate the progress you've made, no matter how incremental.

3.3 Be Kind to Yourself

Health journeys are often filled with ups and downs. Be gentle with yourself when things don't go as planned. Self-compassion is a powerful tool in maintaining motivation and overall well-being. Avoid self-criticism and focus on getting back on track rather than dwelling on past mistakes.

3.4 The Power of Resilience

Through resilience, you can face any obstacles that arise along the way. Resilience allows you to bounce back from challenges and keep moving forward. Remember that the journey is as important as the destination and that setbacks can teach valuable lessons.

Conclusion

In this final chapter, the reader is reminded that taking charge of one's health is an ongoing journey, not a fixed destination. Armed with the knowledge from the book and a personalized health action plan, readers are encouraged to embrace every part of their wellness journey with determination, resilience, and flexibility. This is not about perfection but consistently making choices that lead to a healthier, more balanced life.

Health is a lifelong commitment, and with the tools and strategies provided, readers are empowered to take control of their health and live their best lives.

Conclusion

Congratulations on reaching the end of Women's Wellness: Navigating Your Health Journey. By now, you've gained valuable insights into prioritizing and caring for your physical, mental, and emotional well-being. Your journey toward wellness is personal and continuous, requiring commitment, patience, and compassion. Throughout this book, we've explored the multifaceted nature of women's health, addressing everything from nutrition and exercise to stress management and mental health. You now know to make informed decisions, embrace self-care practices, and cultivate a lifestyle that aligns with your goals and values.

Moving Forward with Confidence:

- **Implement What You've Learned**: Start with small, actionable steps to improve your health and well-being. Whether you adjust your daily habits, add a new self-care routine, or learn how to manage stress, every change you make adds up.

- **Listen to Your Body**: Your body is constantly communicating with you. Learn to tune into its signals, respect its boundaries, and take action when needed. Regular check-ins with your health and wellness goals will keep you on track.

- **Stay Empowered**: Women's wellness is about more than just physical health; it's a holistic approach to every part of you. By nurturing your mind, body, and spirit, you empower yourself to live healthier, happier lives.

- **Seek Support When Needed**: Remember that your health journey doesn't have to be solitary; when you need guidance or encouragement, lean on professionals, friends, family, and support groups. In conclusion, Women's Wellness is an ongoing, evolving process. The knowledge you've gained in this book is just the beginning. The power to shape your health and wellness is in your hands. Embrace the journey, trust yourself, and remember that your health is your most valuable asset. Thank you for allowing me to be a part of your health journey. May you continue to navigate your path with strength, grace, and confidence.

Thank You